HUMAN
ANATOMY
AND PHYSIOLOGY

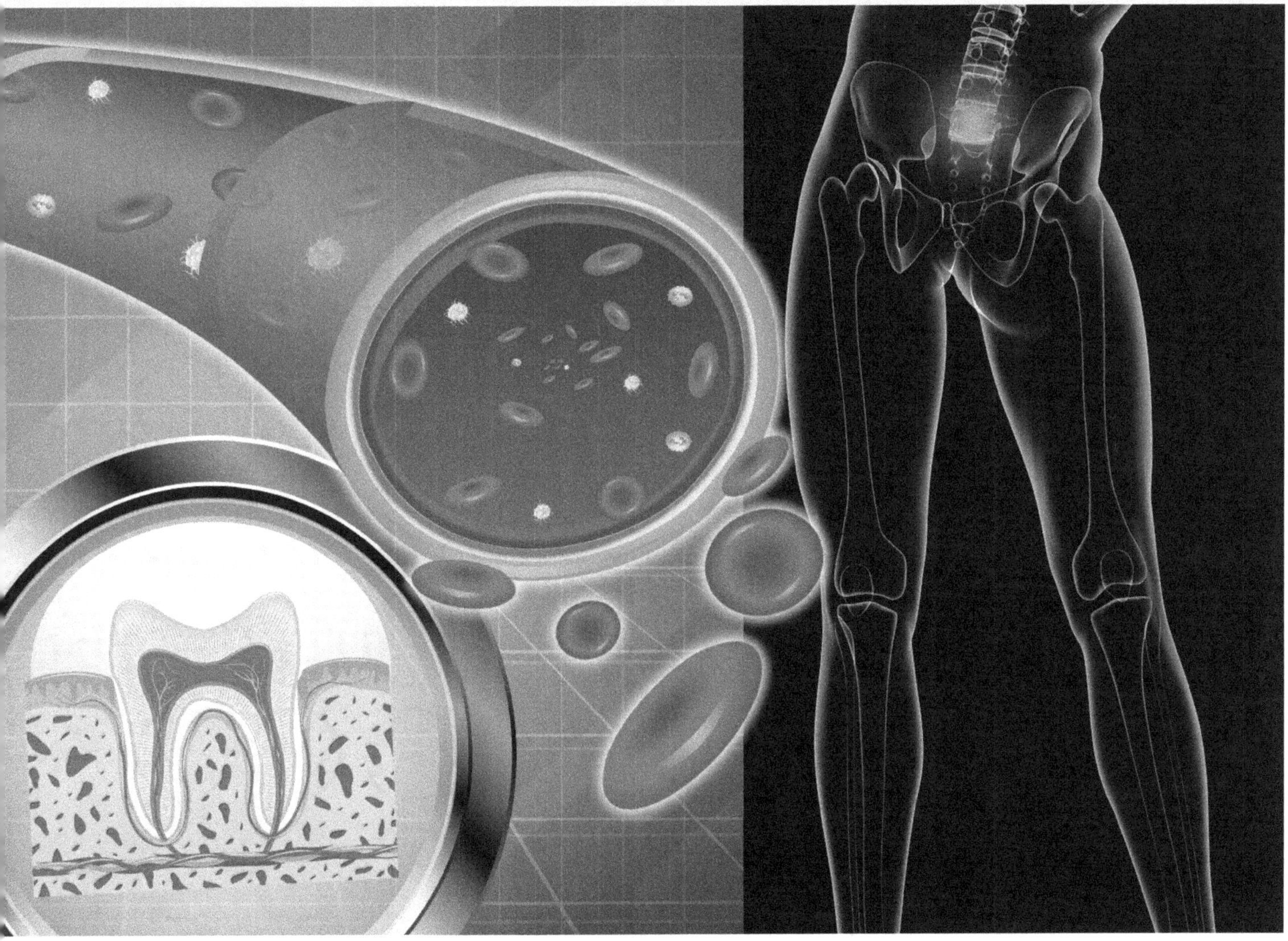

C O L O R I N G   B O O K

COLOR TEST PAGE

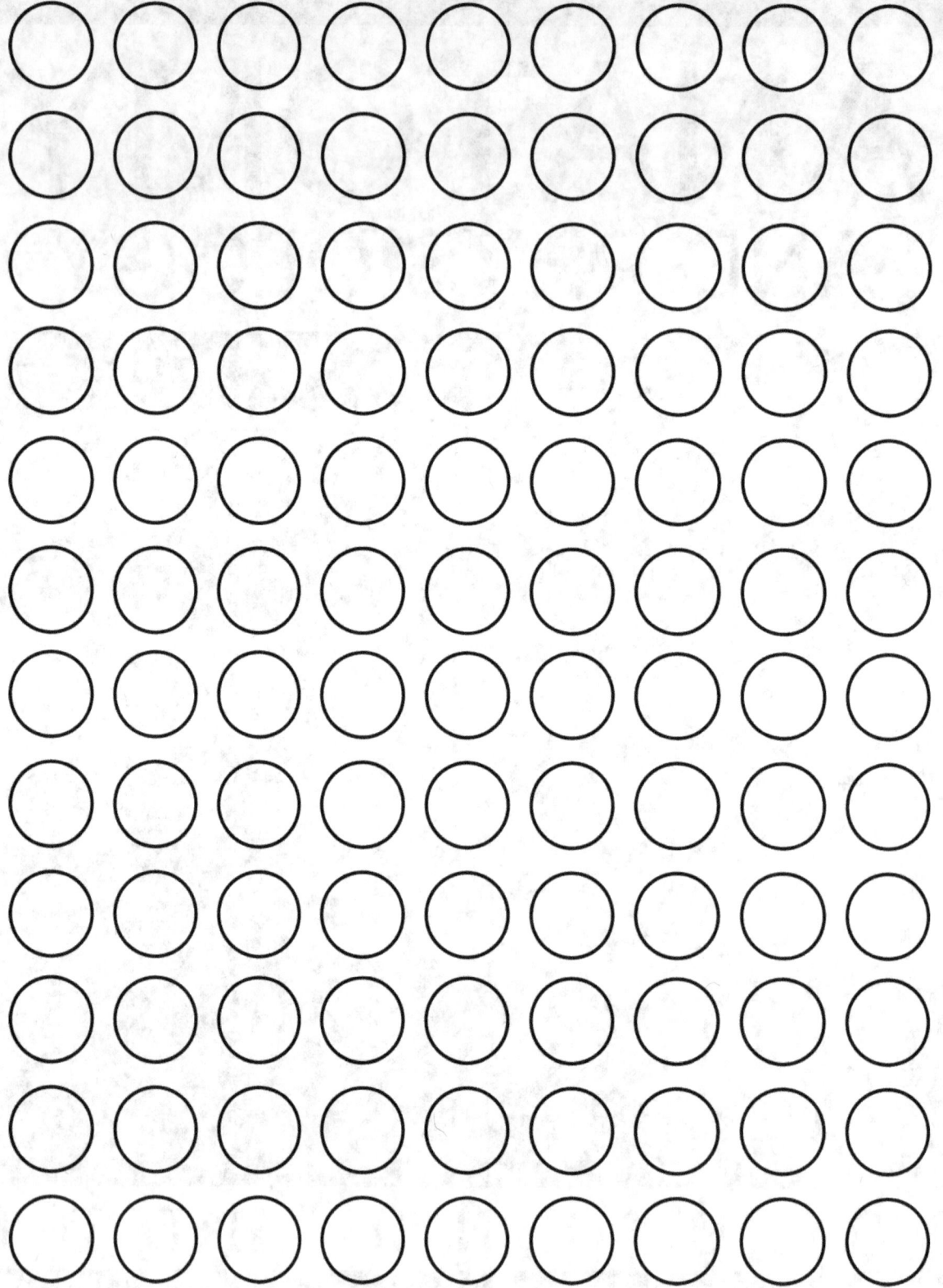

COLOR TEST PAGE

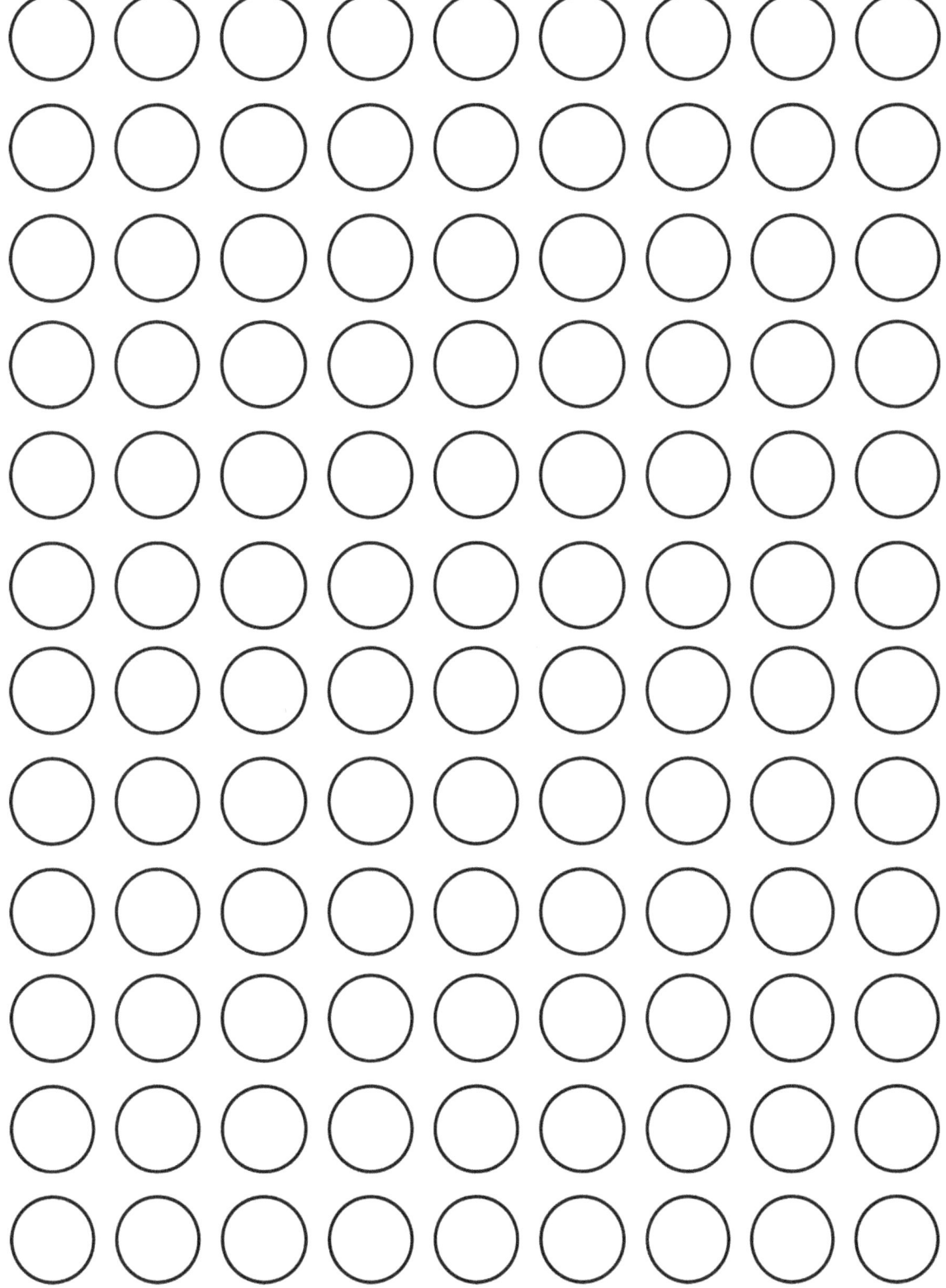

SKULL

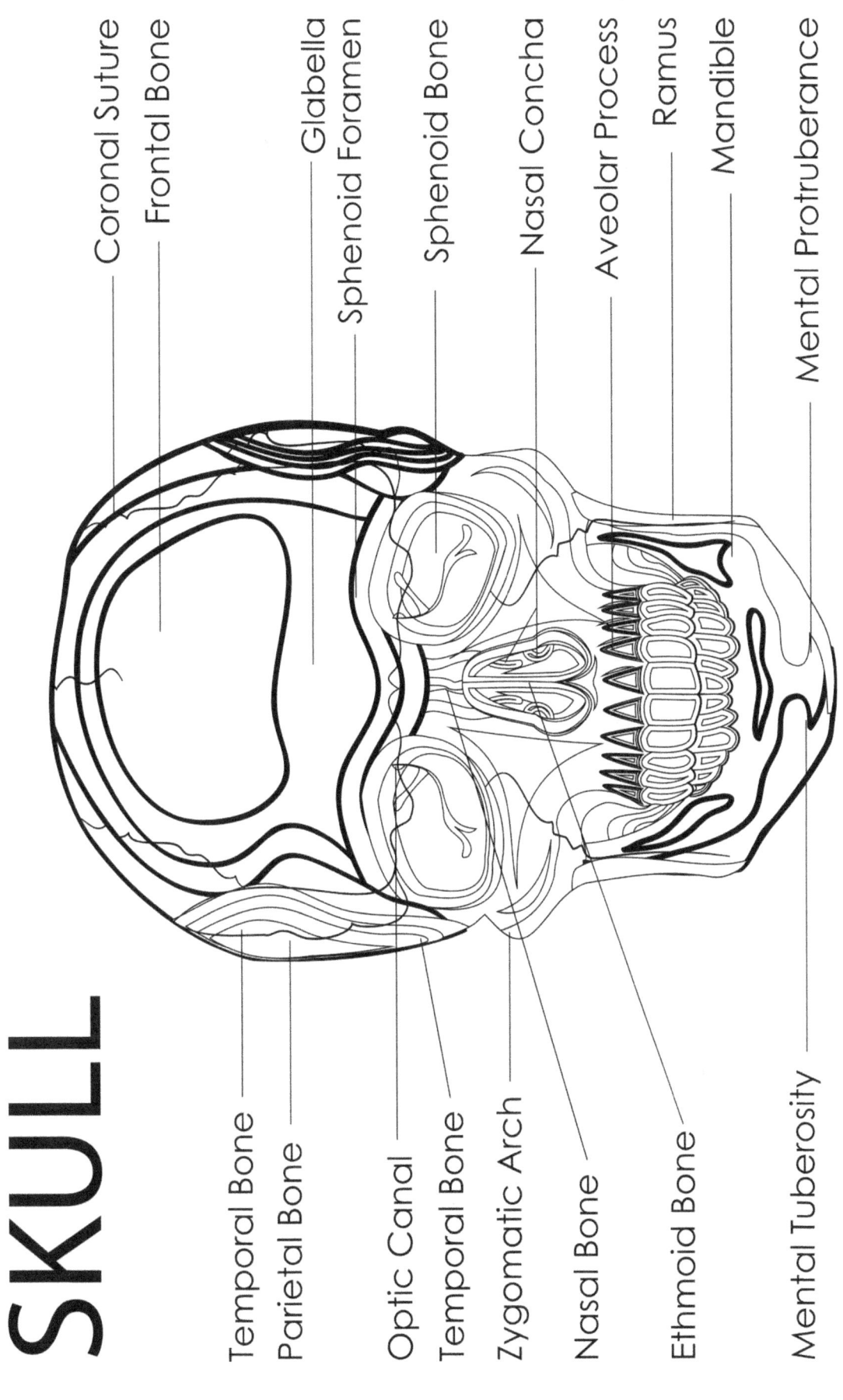

Coronal Suture
Frontal Bone
Glabella
Sphenoid Foramen
Sphenoid Bone
Nasal Concha
Aveolar Process
Ramus
Mandible
Mental Protruberance

Temporal Bone
Parietal Bone
Optic Canal
Temporal Bone
Zygomatic Arch
Nasal Bone
Ethmoid Bone
Mental Tuberosity

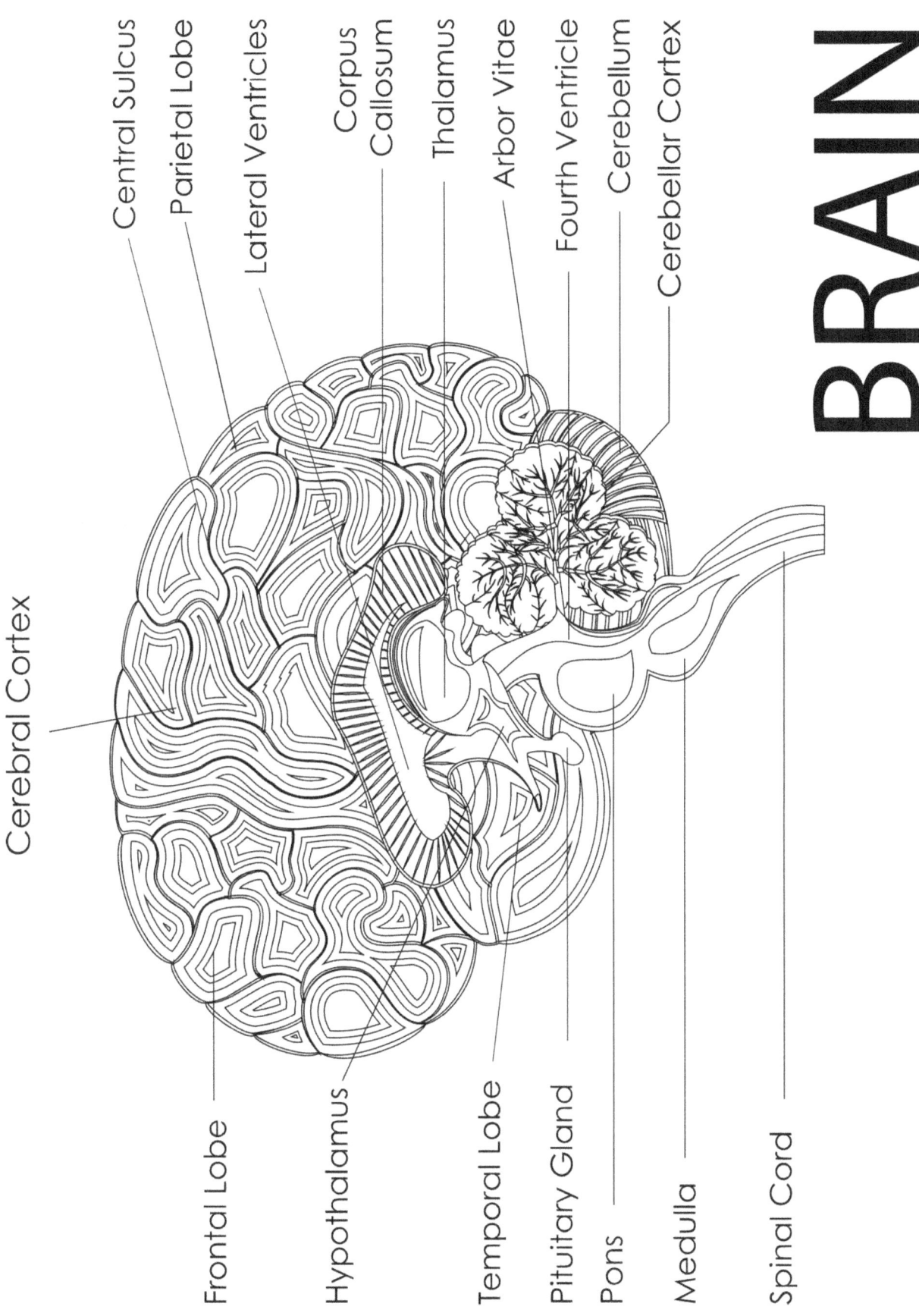

Central Sulcus

Parietal Lobe

Lateral Ventricles

Corpus Callosum

Thalamus

Arbor Vitae

Fourth Ventricle

Cerebellum

Cerebellar Cortex

Cerebral Cortex

Frontal Lobe

Hypothalamus

Temporal Lobe

Pituitary Gland

Pons

Medulla

Spinal Cord

BRAIN

EYE

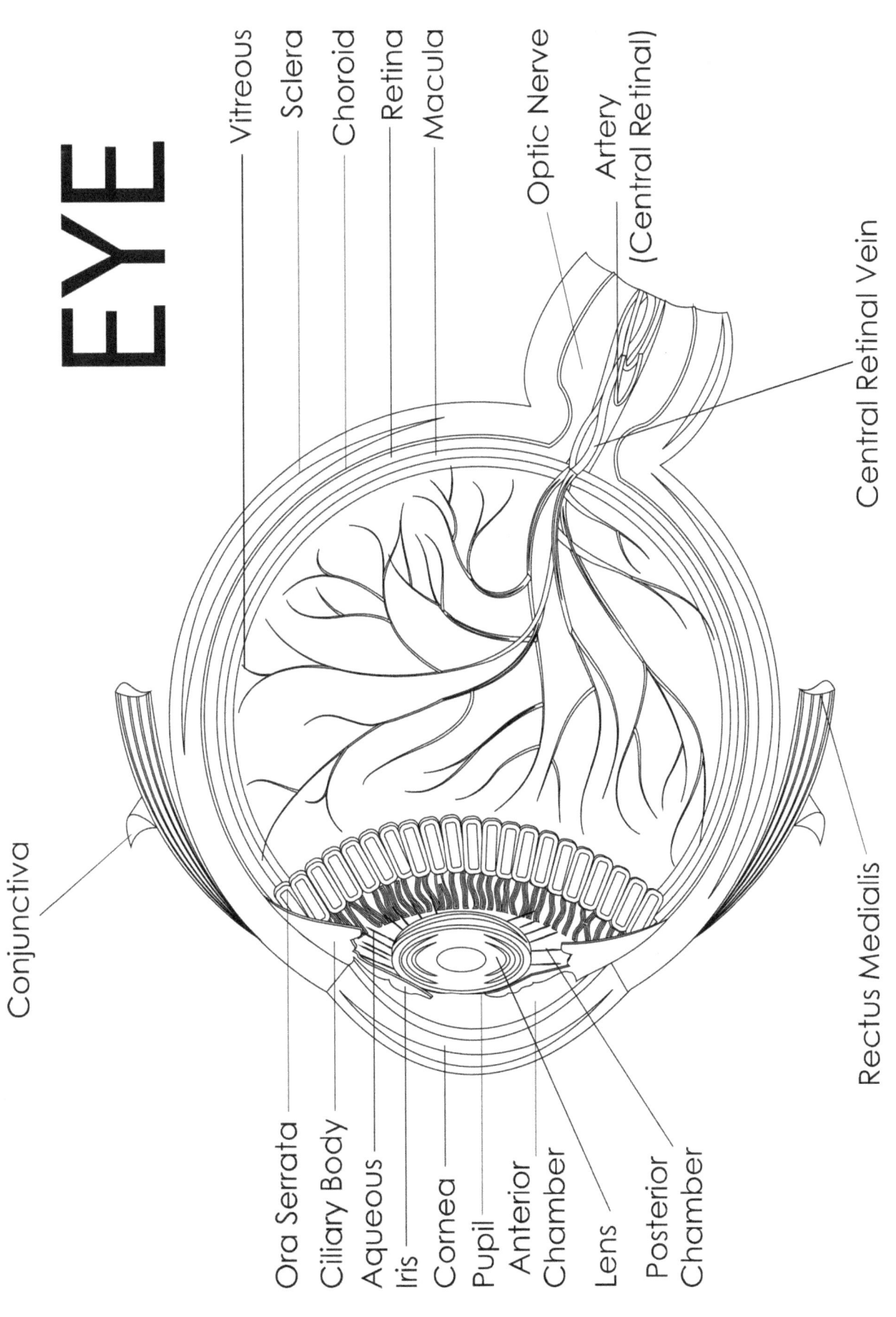

Vitreous

Sclera

Choroid

Retina

Macula

Optic Nerve

Artery
(Central Retinal)

Central Retinal Vein

Conjunctiva

Ora Serrata

Ciliary Body

Aqueous

Iris

Cornea

Pupil

Anterior
Chamber

Lens

Posterior
Chamber

Rectus Medialis

Central Incisor
Lateral Incisor
Canine
Premolars
Molars

Soft Palate

Tonsil

Tongue

Lingual Frenulum

Sublingual Papilla

Vestibule

Inferior Lip

Superior Lip
Superior Labial Frenulum
Palatine Raphe
Hard Palate

Palatoglossal Arch

Palatopharyngeal Arch

Uvula

Oropharynx

Gingivae (gums)

Inferior Labial Frenulum

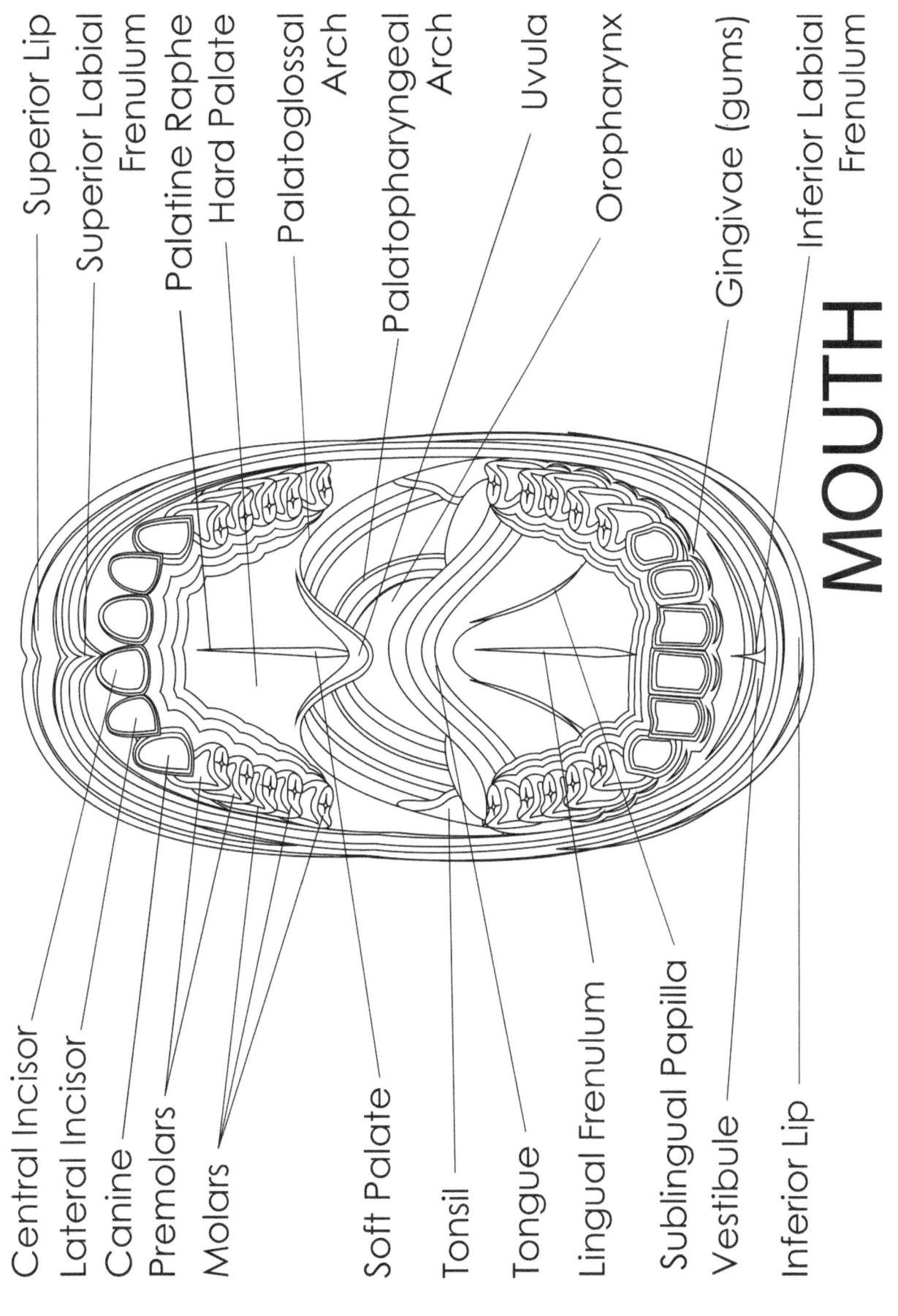

MOUTH

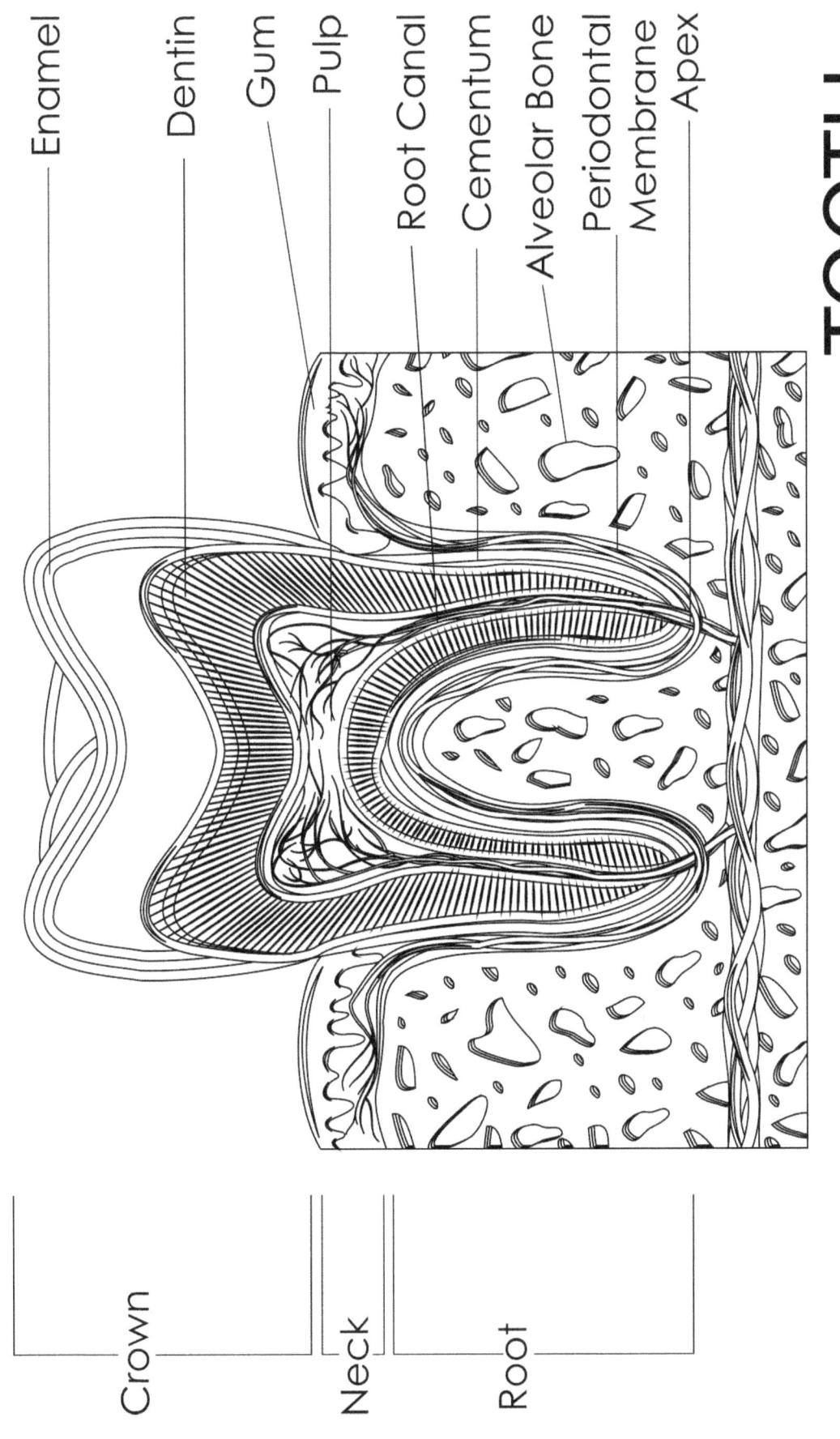

Enamel

Dentin

Gum

Pulp

Root Canal

Cementum

Alveolar Bone

Periodontal
Membrane

Apex

Crown

Neck

Root

TOOTH

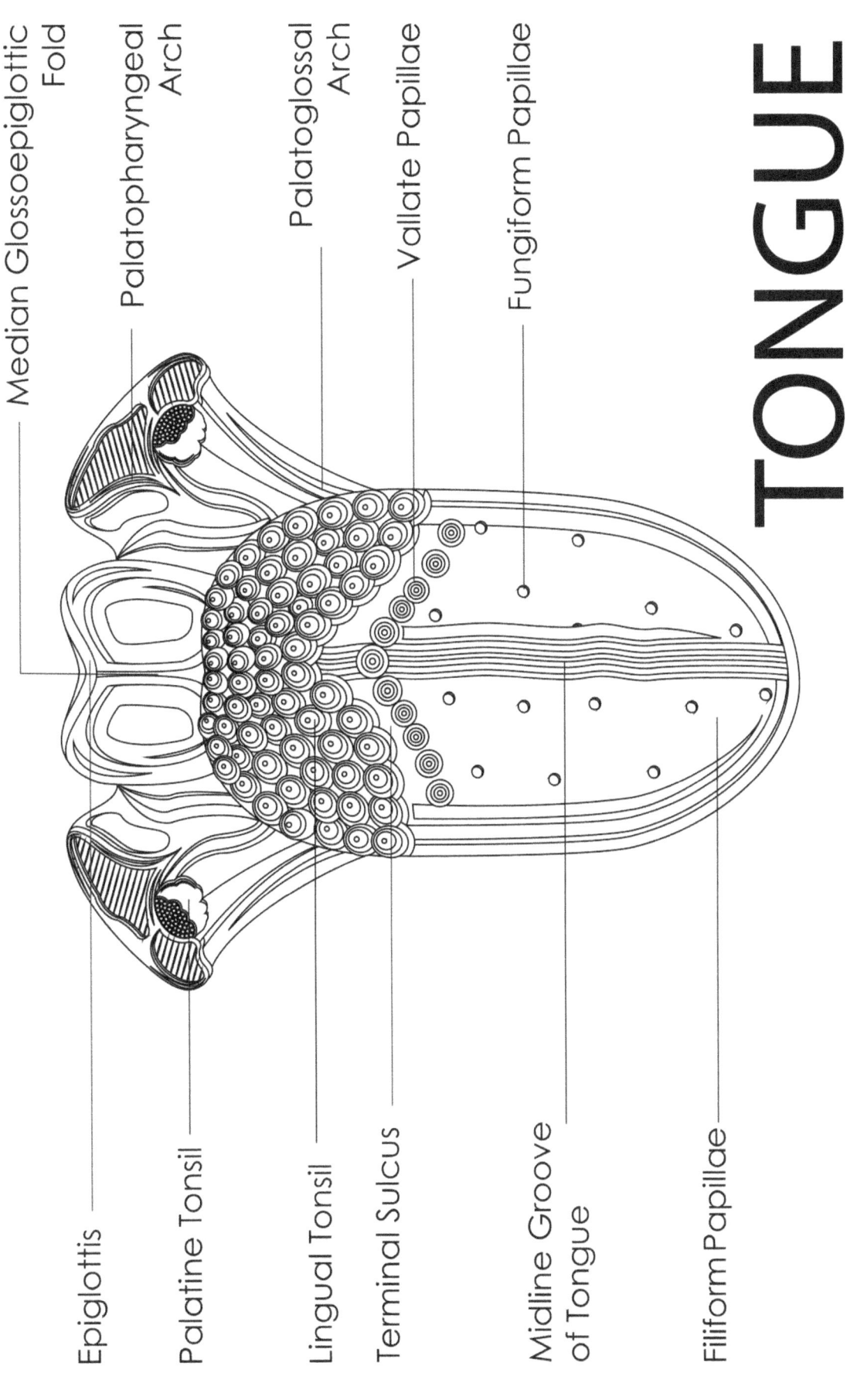

Median Glossoepiglottic
Fold

Palatopharyngeal
Arch

Palatoglossal
Arch

Vallate Papillae

Fungiform Papillae

Epiglottis

Palatine Tonsil

Lingual Tonsil

Terminal Sulcus

Midline Groove
of Tongue

Filiform Papillae

TONGUE

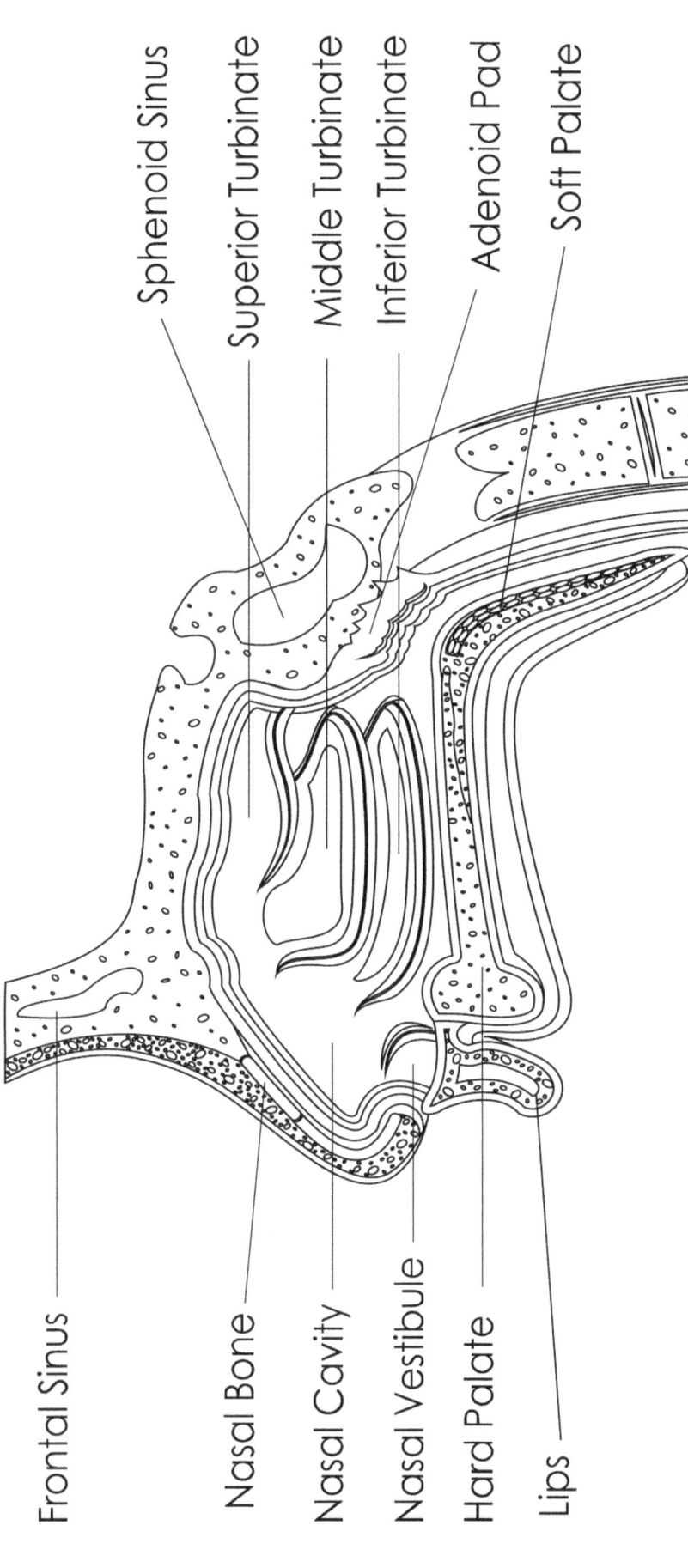

Frontal Sinus

Nasal Bone

Nasal Cavity

Nasal Vestibule

Hard Palate

Lips

Sphenoid Sinus

Superior Turbinate

Middle Turbinate

Inferior Turbinate

Adenoid Pad

Soft Palate

NOSE

THROAT

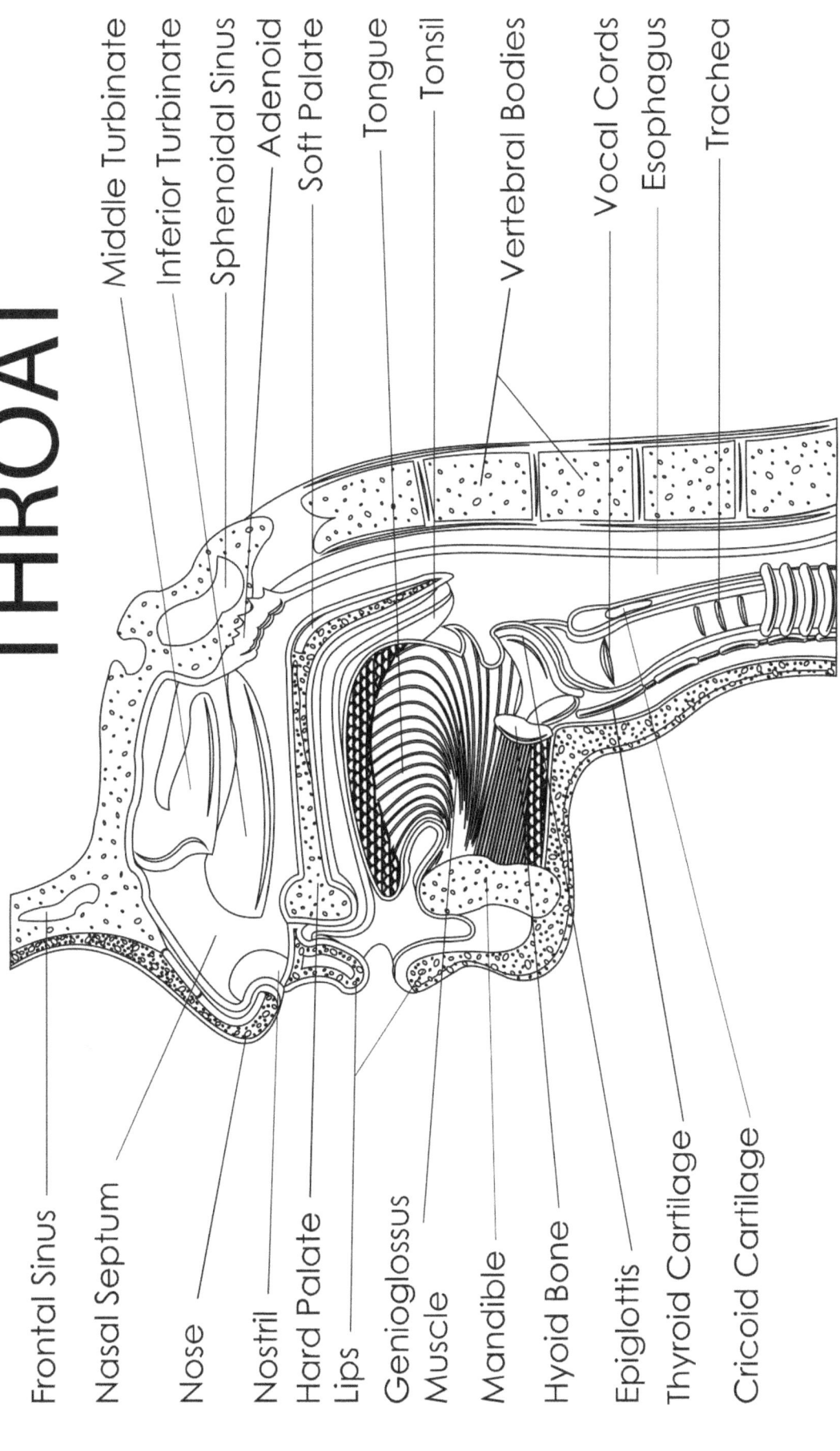

Frontal Sinus

Nasal Septum

Nose

Nostril

Hard Palate

Lips

Genioglossus
Muscle

Mandible

Hyoid Bone

Epiglottis

Thyroid Cartilage

Cricoid Cartilage

Middle Turbinate

Inferior Turbinate

Sphenoidal Sinus

Adenoid

Soft Palate

Tongue

Tonsil

Vertebral Bodies

Vocal Cords

Esophagus

Trachea

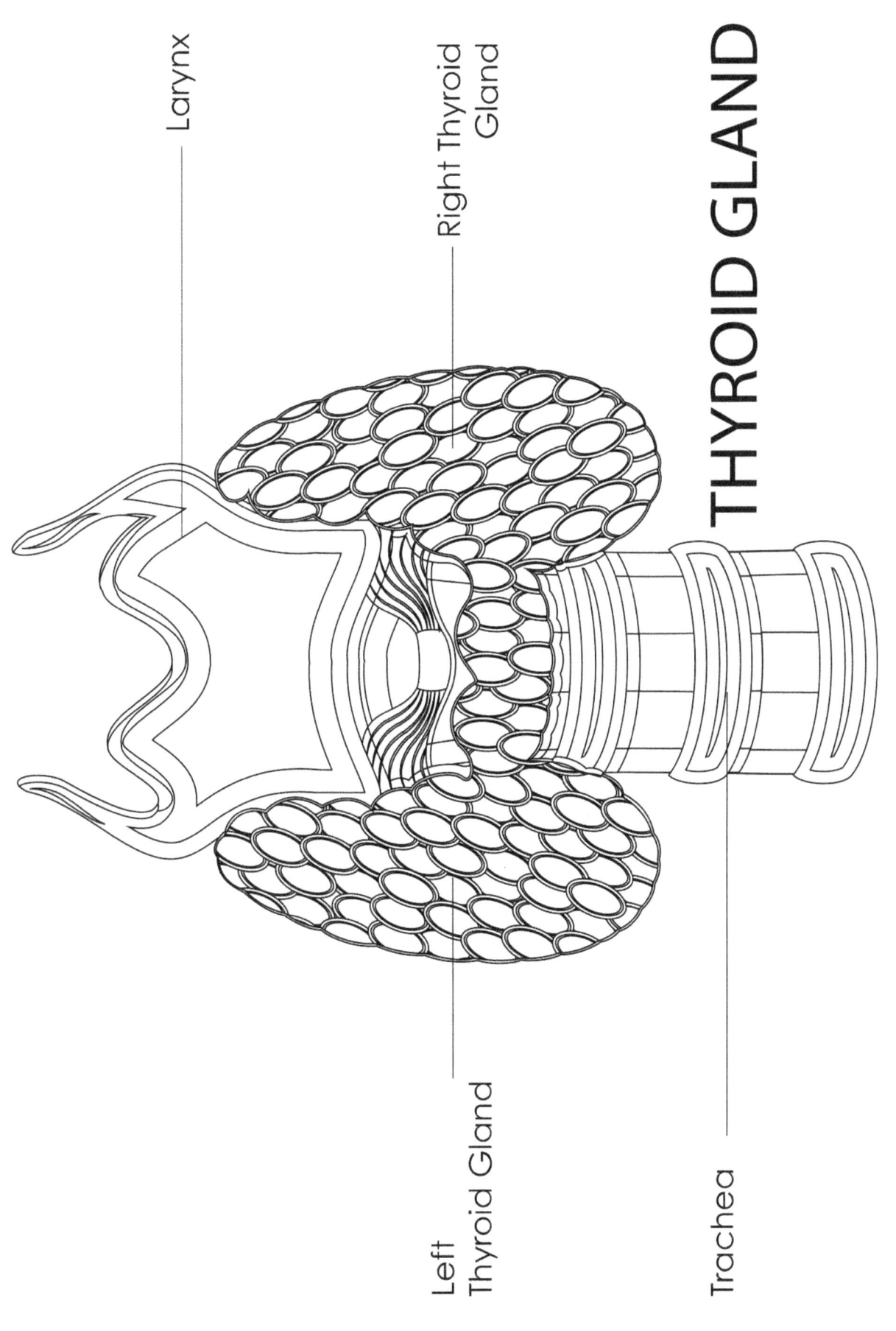

Larynx

Right Thyroid
Gland

Left
Thyroid Gland

Trachea

THYROID GLAND

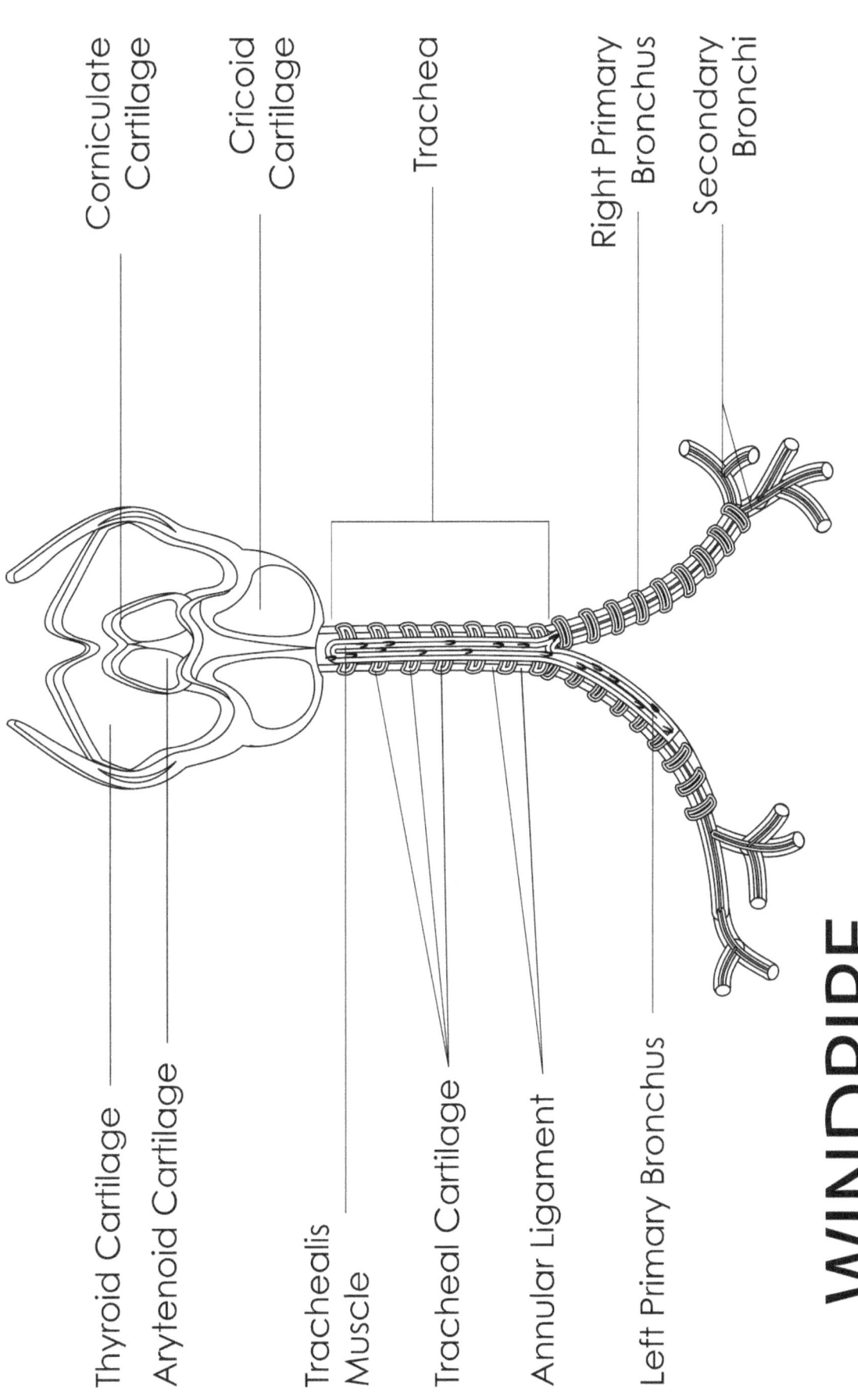

Corniculate
Cartilage

Cricoid
Cartilage

Trachea

Right Primary
Bronchus

Secondary
Bronchi

Thyroid Cartilage

Arytenoid Cartilage

Trachealis
Muscle

Tracheal Cartilage

Annular Ligament

Left Primary Bronchus

WINDPIPE

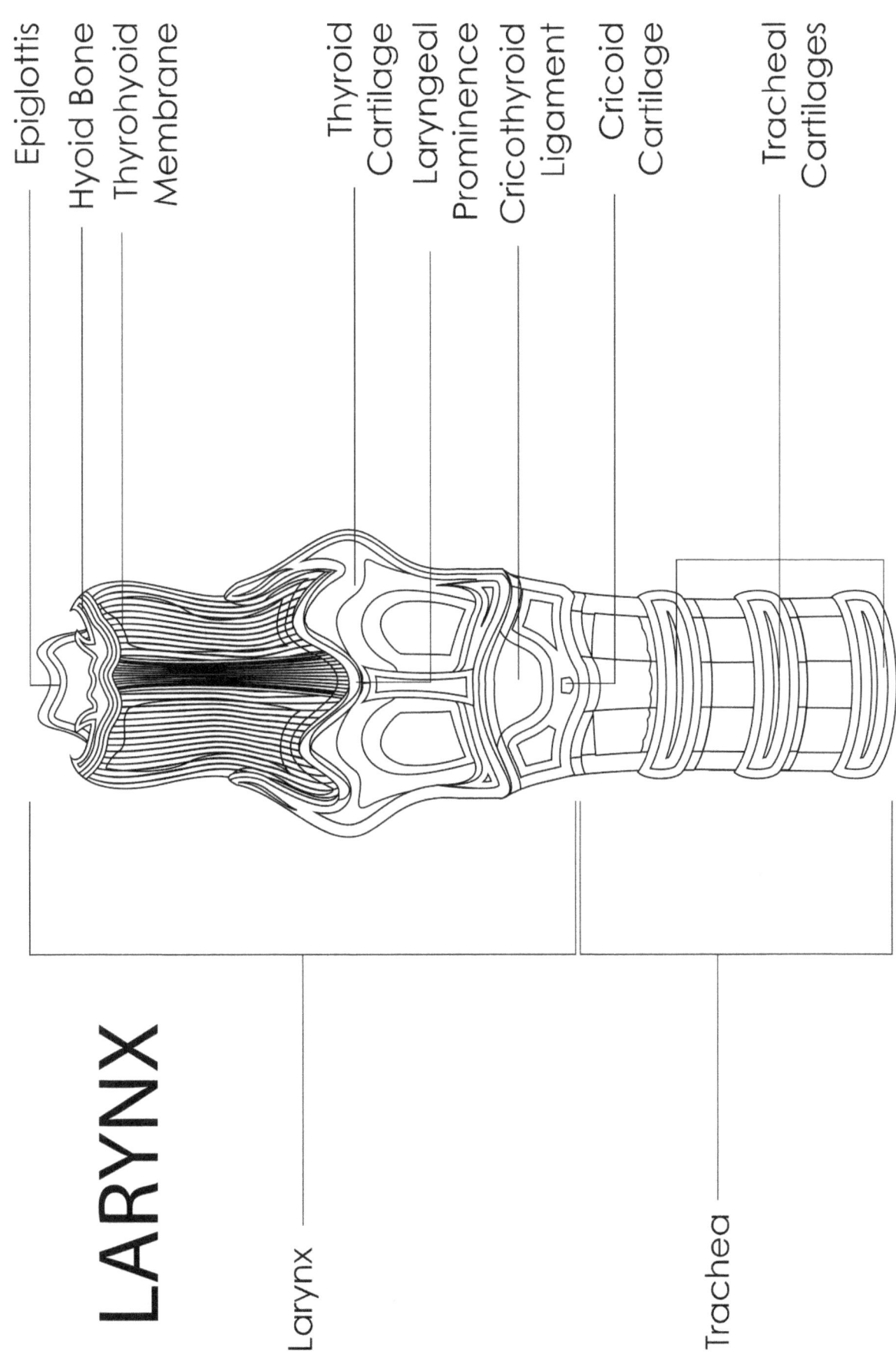

LARYNX

Epiglottis

Hyoid Bone

Thyrohyoid Membrane

Thyroid Cartilage

Laryngeal Prominence

Cricothyroid Ligament

Cricoid Cartilage

Tracheal Cartilages

Larynx

Trachea

EAR

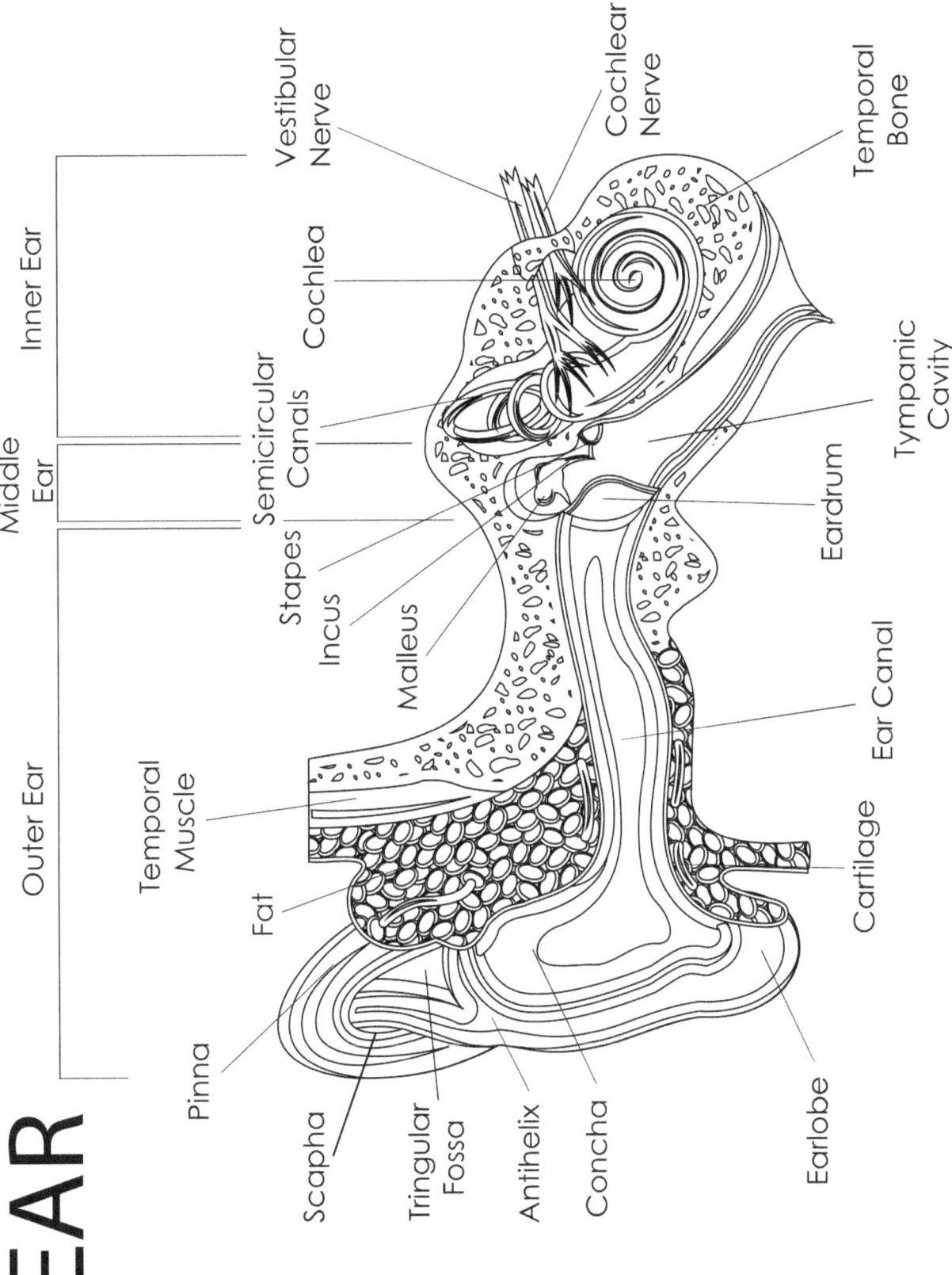

Outer Ear

Middle Ear

Inner Ear

Vestibular Nerve

Cochlear Nerve

Temporal Bone

Cochlea

Semicircular Canals

Stapes

Incus

Malleus

Temporal Muscle

Fat

Tympanic Cavity

Eardrum

Ear Canal

Cartilage

Pinna

Scapha

Tringular Fossa

Antihelix

Concha

Earlobe

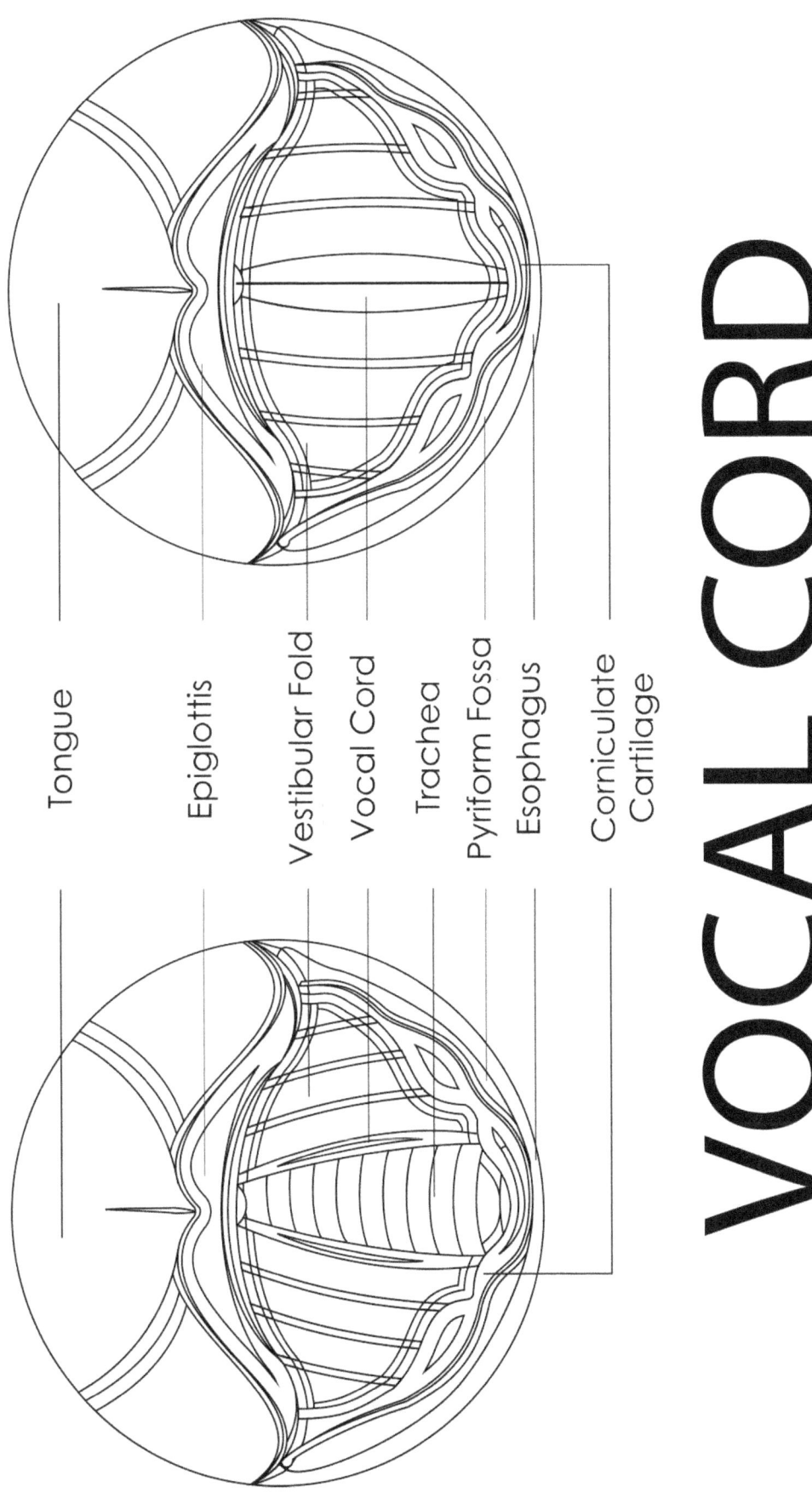

Tongue

Epiglottis

Vestibular Fold

Vocal Cord

Trachea

Pyriform Fossa

Esophagus

Corniculate
Cartilage

VOCAL CORD

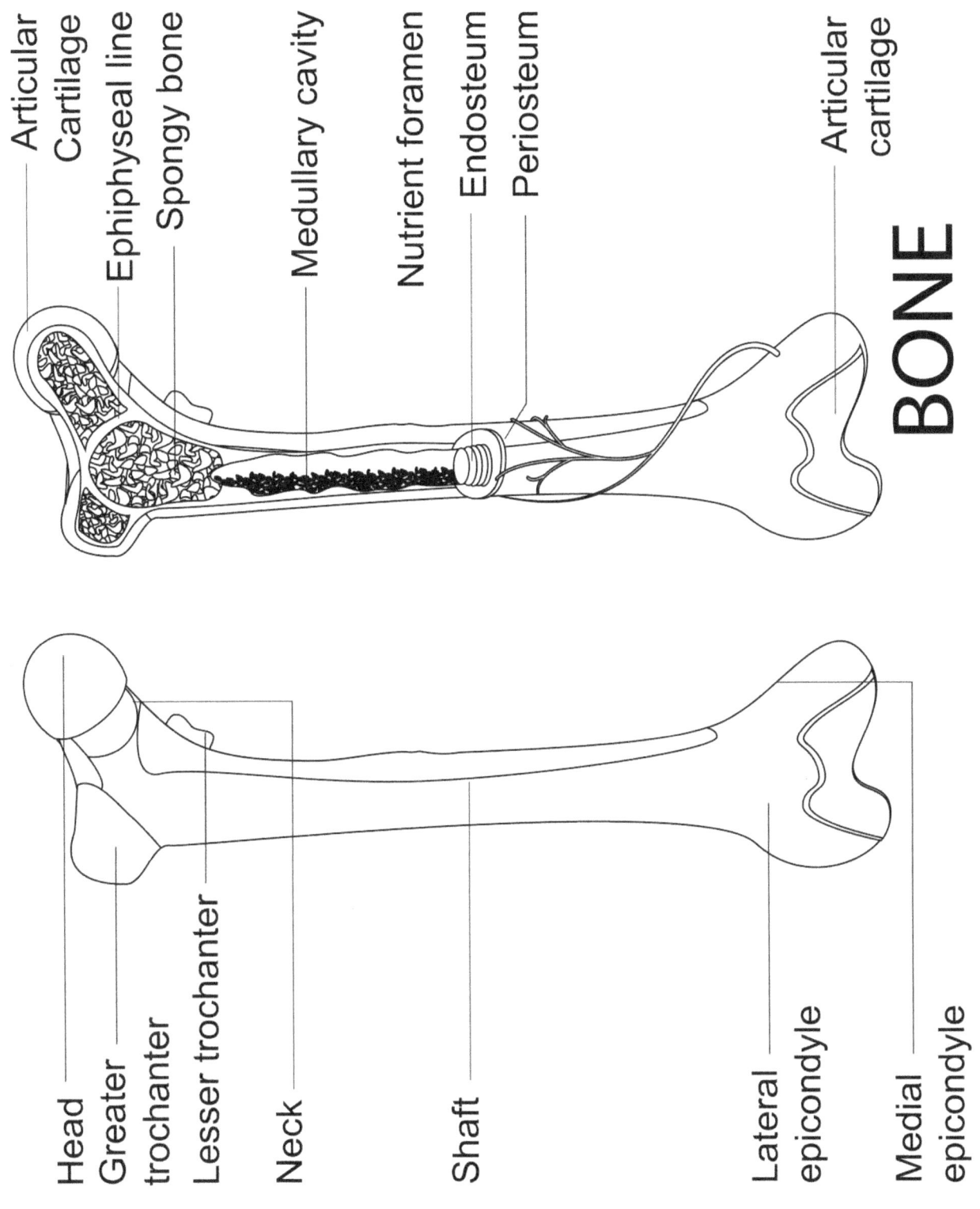

Articular
Cartilage

Ephiphyseal line
Spongy bone

Medullary cavity

Nutrient foramen

Endosteum
Periosteum

Articular
cartilage

BONE

Head
Greater
trochanter
Lesser trochanter

Neck

Shaft

Lateral
epicondyle

Medial
epicondyle

TEETH

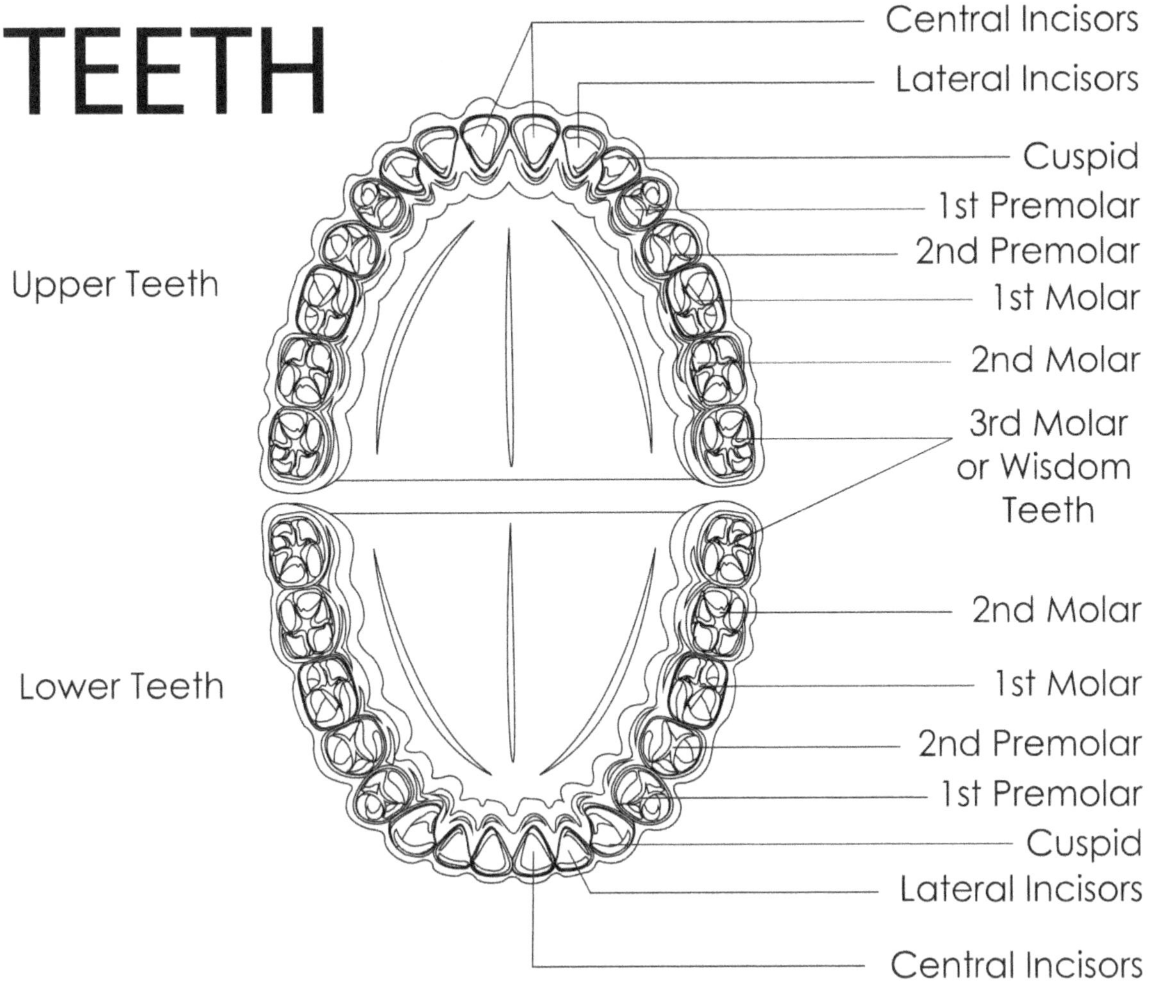

Upper Teeth

Central Incisors
Lateral Incisors
Cuspid
1st Premolar
2nd Premolar
1st Molar
2nd Molar
3rd Molar or Wisdom Teeth
2nd Molar
1st Molar
2nd Premolar
1st Premolar
Cuspid
Lateral Incisors
Central Incisors

Lower Teeth

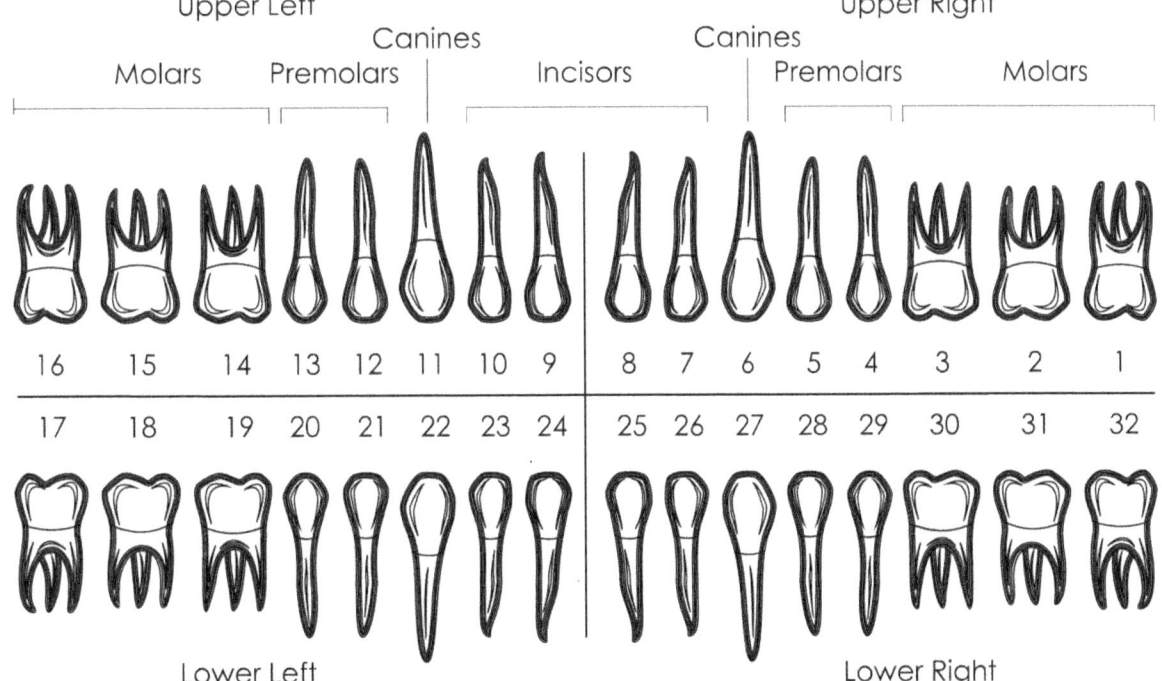

Upper Left								Upper Right							
Molars			Premolars		Canines	Incisors			Canines	Premolars		Molars			
16	15	14	13	12	11	10	9	8	7	6	5	4	3	2	1
17	18	19	20	21	22	23	24	25	26	27	28	29	30	31	32
Lower Left								Lower Right							

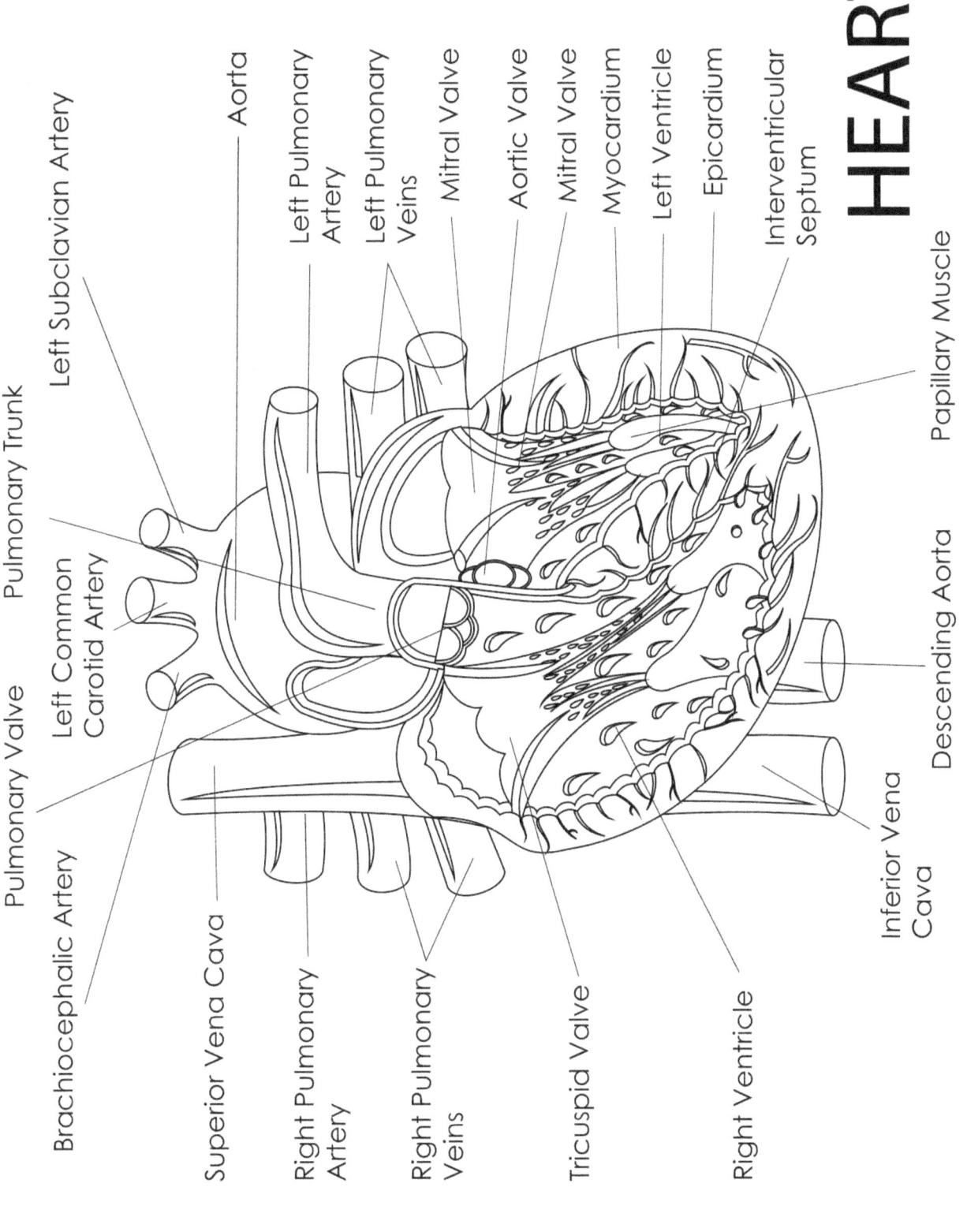

Brachiocephalic Artery

Pulmonary Valve   Pulmonary Trunk

Left Common
Carotid Artery

Left Subclavian Artery

Aorta

Left Pulmonary
Artery

Left Pulmonary
Veins

Mitral Valve

Aortic Valve

Mitral Valve

Myocardium

Left Ventricle

Epicardium

Interventricular
Septum

HEART

Papillary Muscle

Descending Aorta

Inferior Vena
Cava

Right Ventricle

Tricuspid Valve

Right Pulmonary
Veins

Right Pulmonary
Artery

Superior Vena Cava

LUNGS

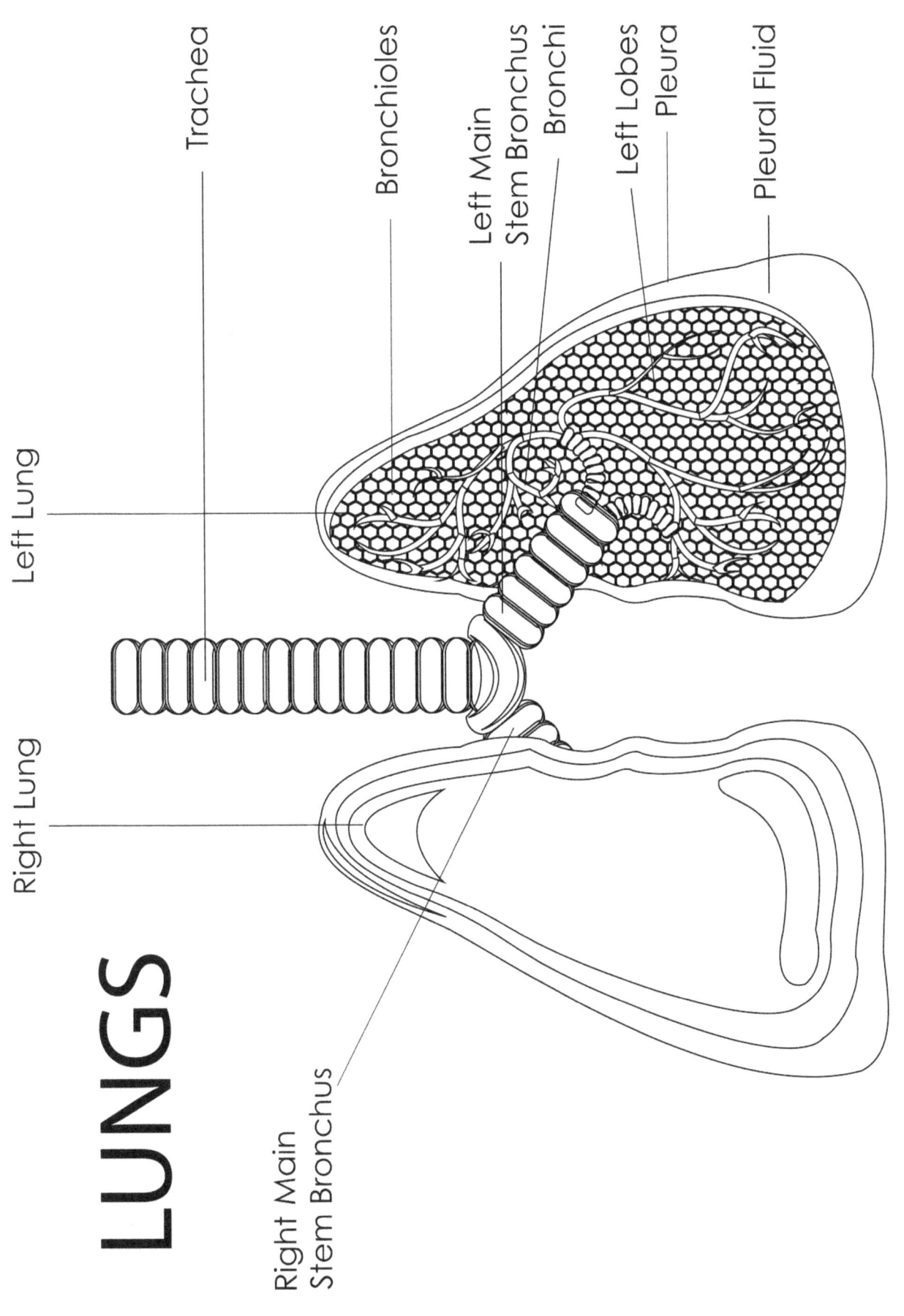

Trachea

Bronchioles

Left Main
Stem Bronchus

Bronchi

Left Lobes

Pleura

Pleural Fluid

Left Lung

Right Lung

Right Main
Stem Bronchus

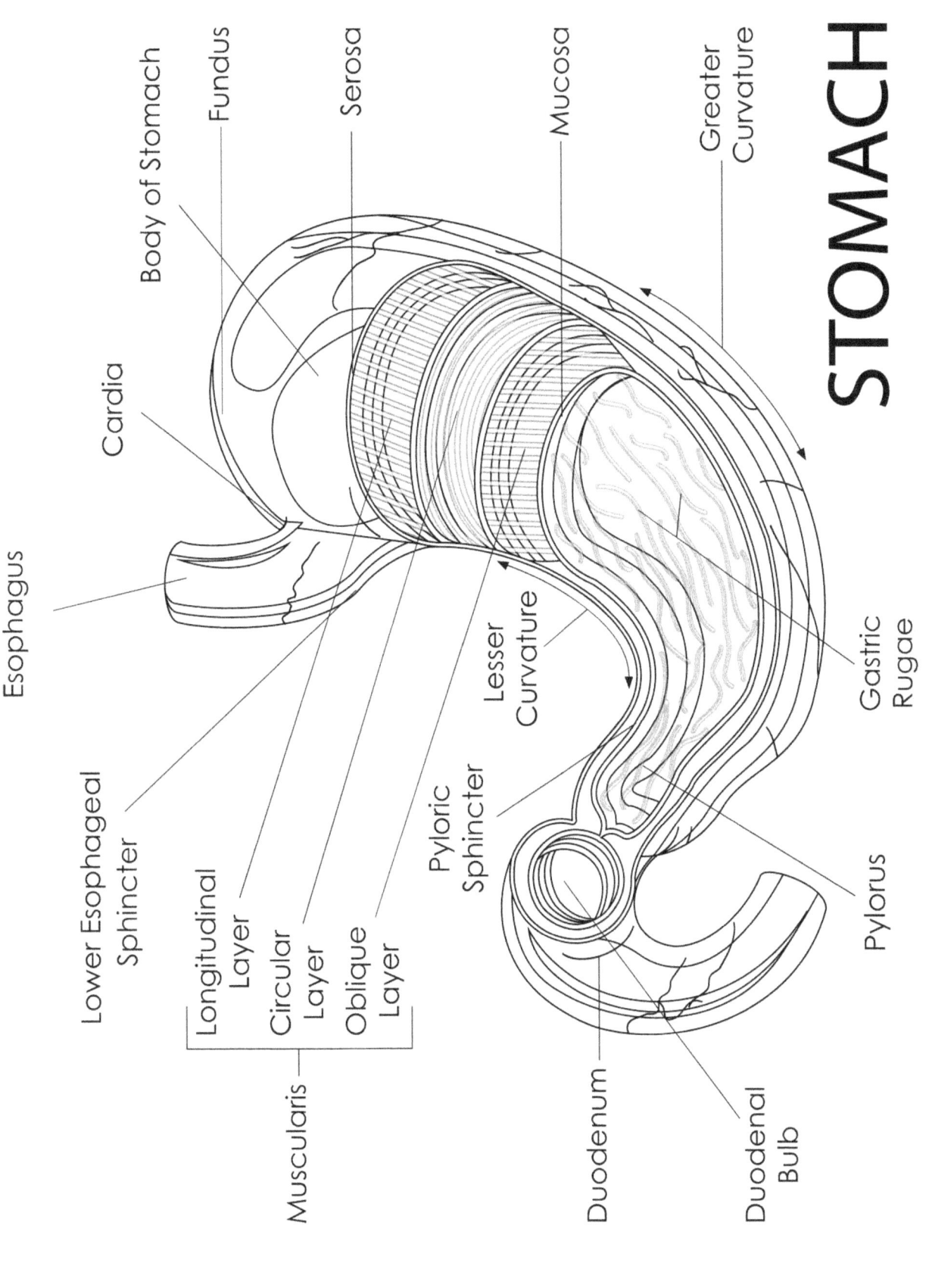

Esophagus

Fundus

Body of Stomach

Cardia

Serosa

Mucosa

Greater Curature

Lower Esophageal Sphincter

Muscularis

Longitudinal Layer

Circular Layer

Oblique Layer

Lesser Curvature

Pyloric Sphincter

Gastric Rugae

Duodenum

Duodenal Bulb

Pylorus

STOMACH

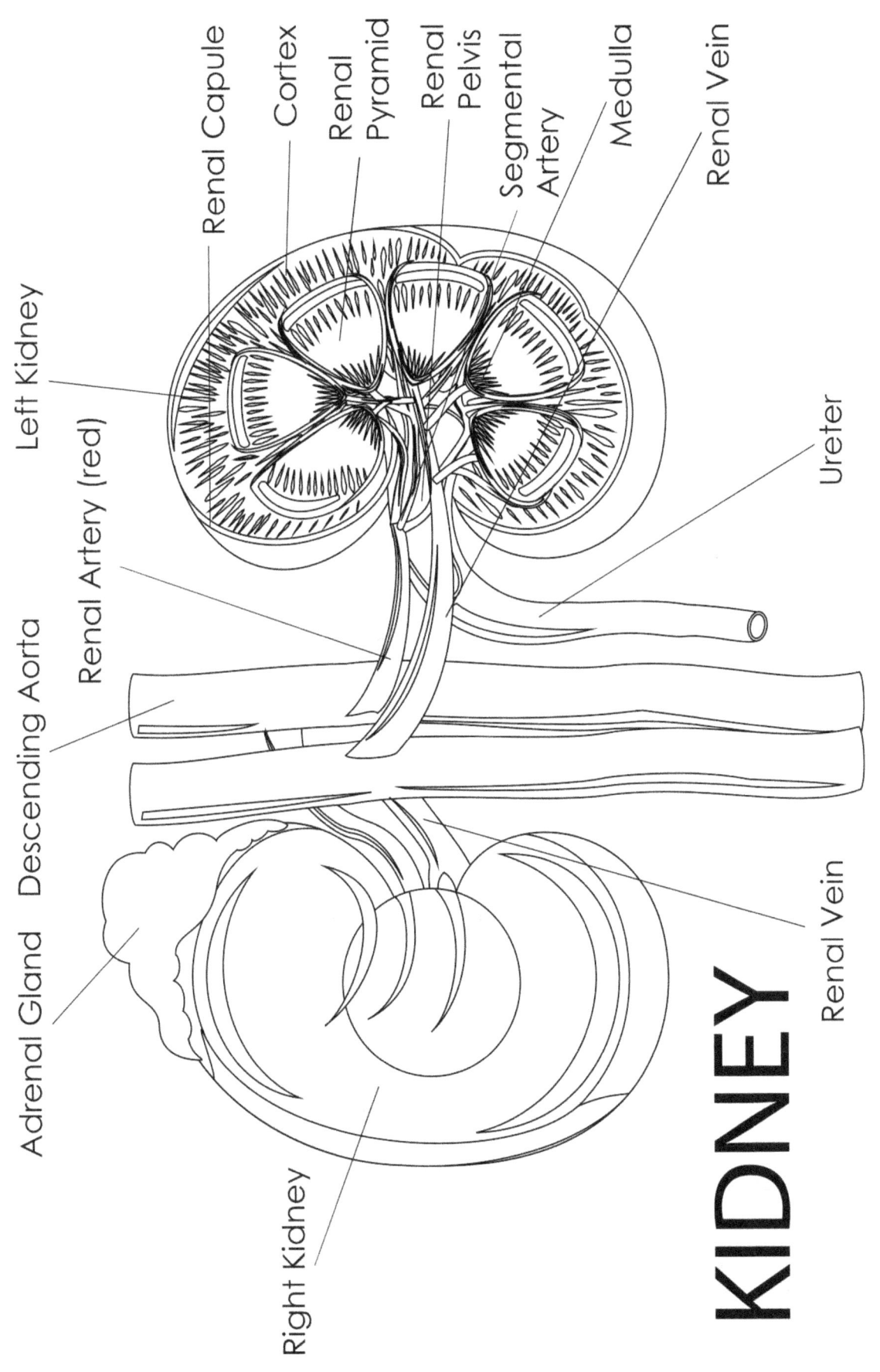

Renal Capule

Cortex

Renal Pyramid

Renal Pelvis

Segmental Artery

Medulla

Renal Vein

Left Kidney

Renal Artery (red)

Descending Aorta

Adrenal Gland

Right Kidney

Ureter

Renal Vein

KIDNEY

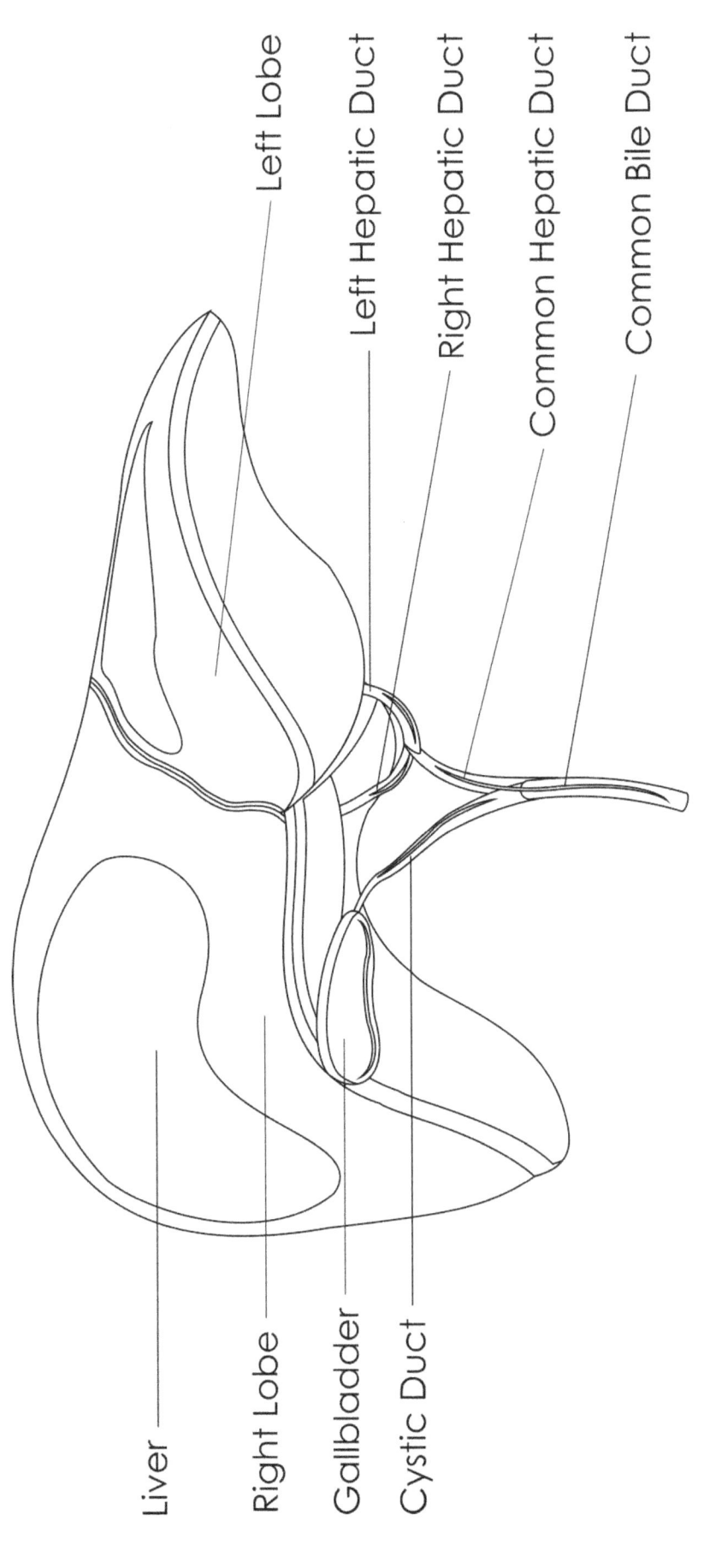

Left Lobe

Left Hepatic Duct

Right Hepatic Duct

Common Hepatic Duct

Common Bile Duct

Liver

Right Lobe

Gallbladder

Cystic Duct

LIVER

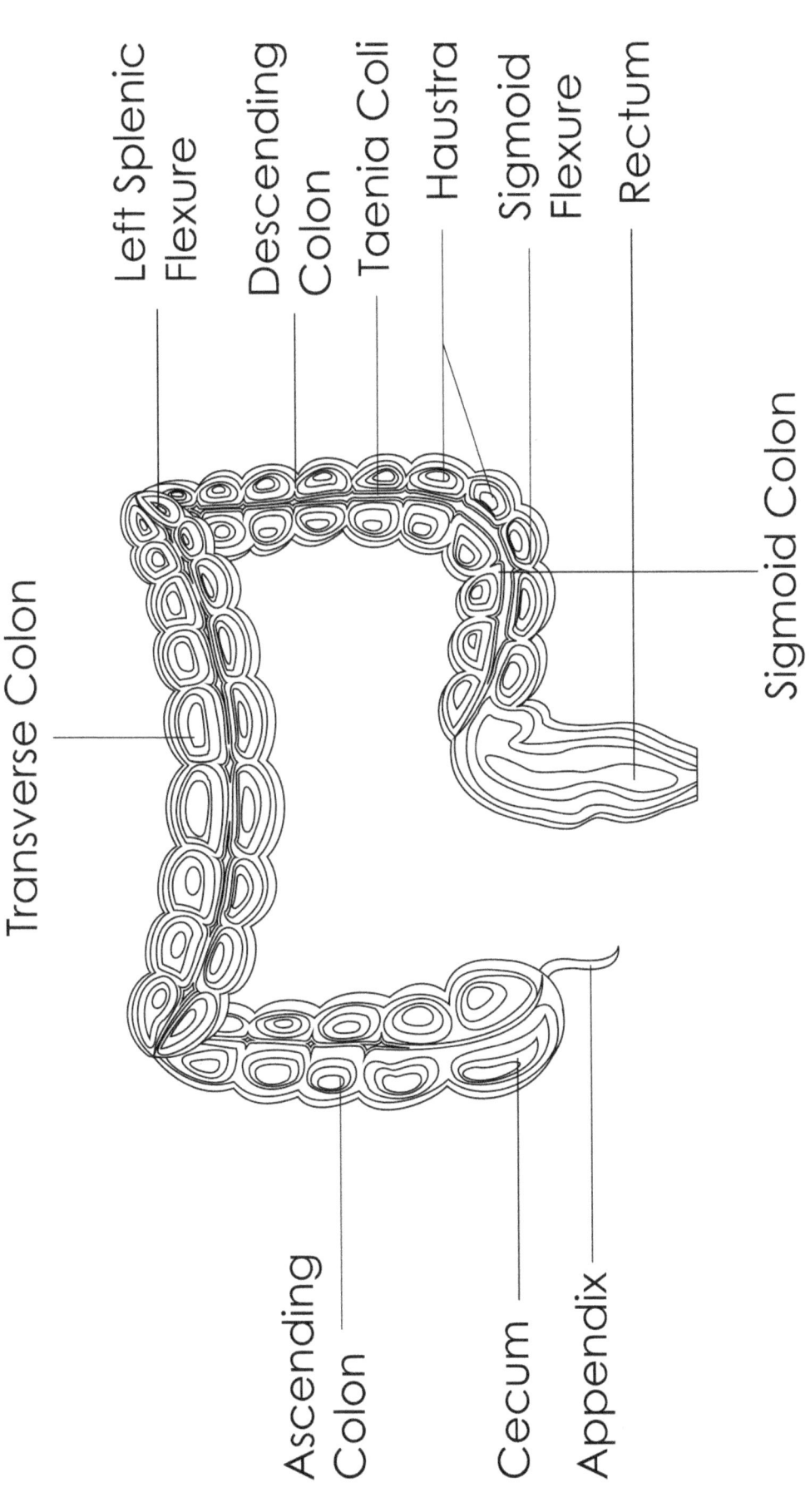

Left Splenic
Flexure

Descending
Colon

Taenia Coli

Haustra

Sigmoid
Flexure

Rectum

Transverse Colon

Sigmoid Colon

Ascending
Colon

Cecum

Appendix

LARGE INTESTINE

FLOW OF BLOOD

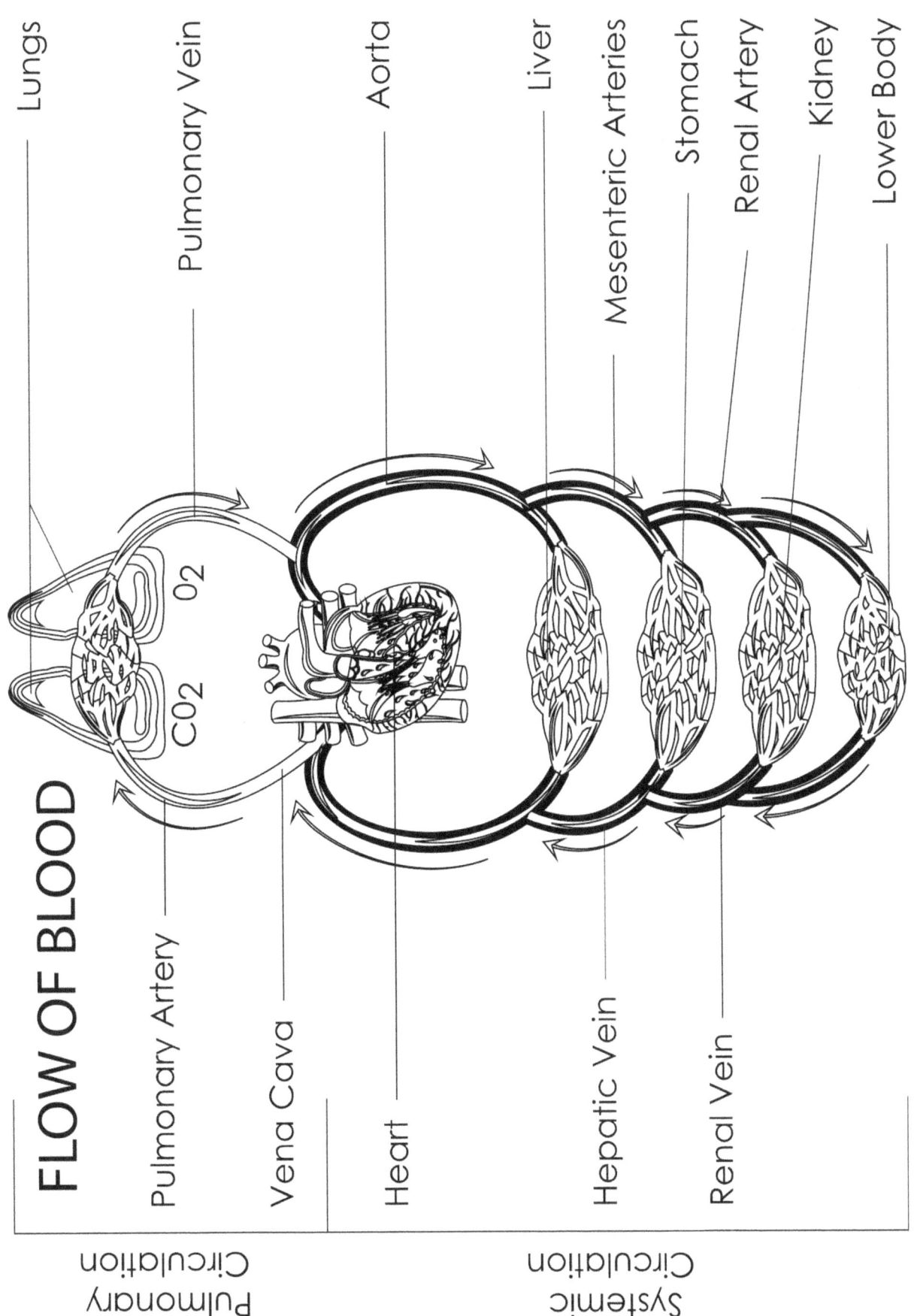

Lungs

Pulmonary Vein

Aorta

Liver

Mesenteric Arteries

Stomach

Renal Artery

Kidney

Lower Body

Pulmonary Artery

Vena Cava

Heart

Hepatic Vein

Renal Vein

O_2

CO_2

Pulmonary Circulation

Systemic Circulation

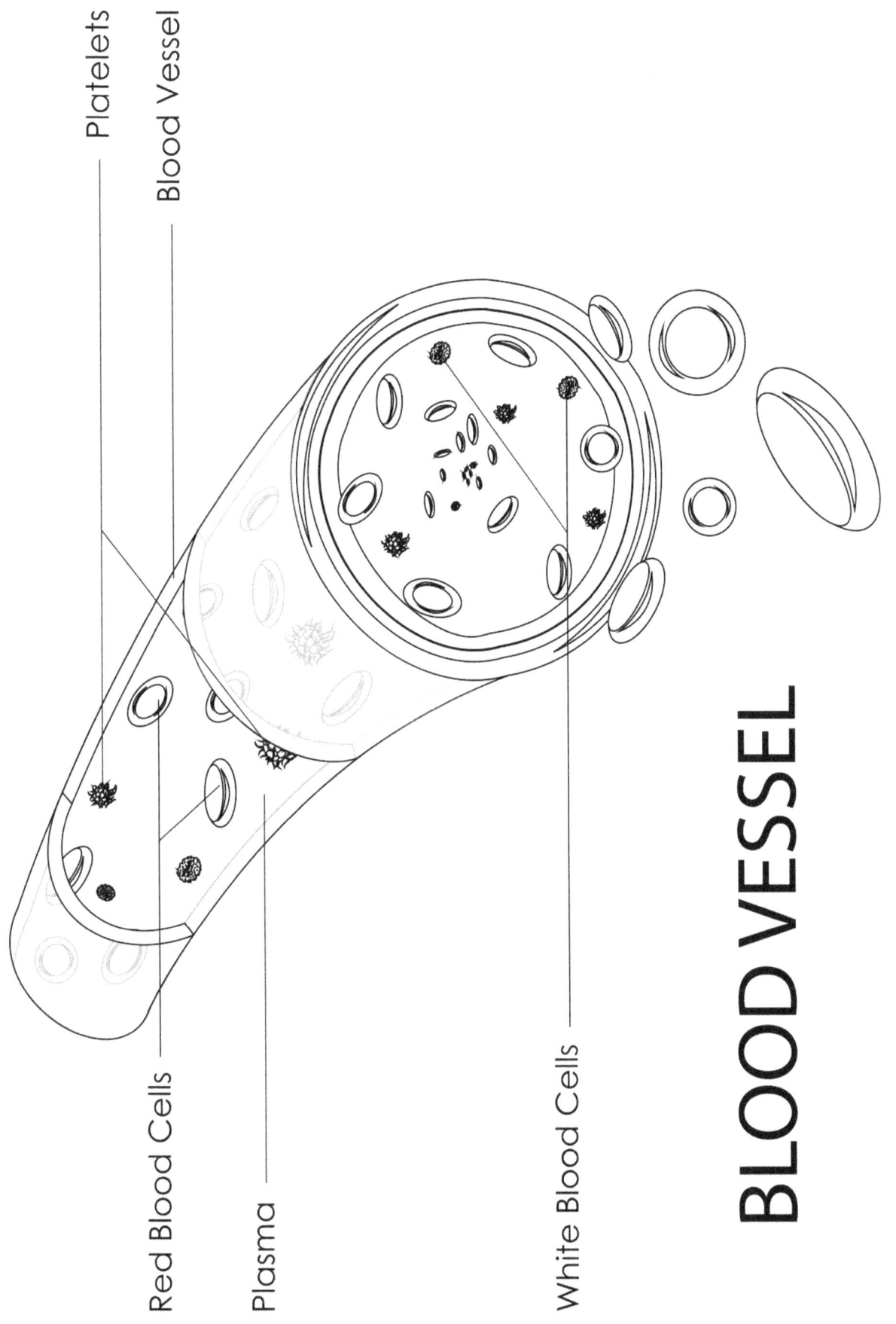

Platelets

Blood Vessel

Red Blood Cells

Plasma

White Blood Cells

BLOOD VESSEL

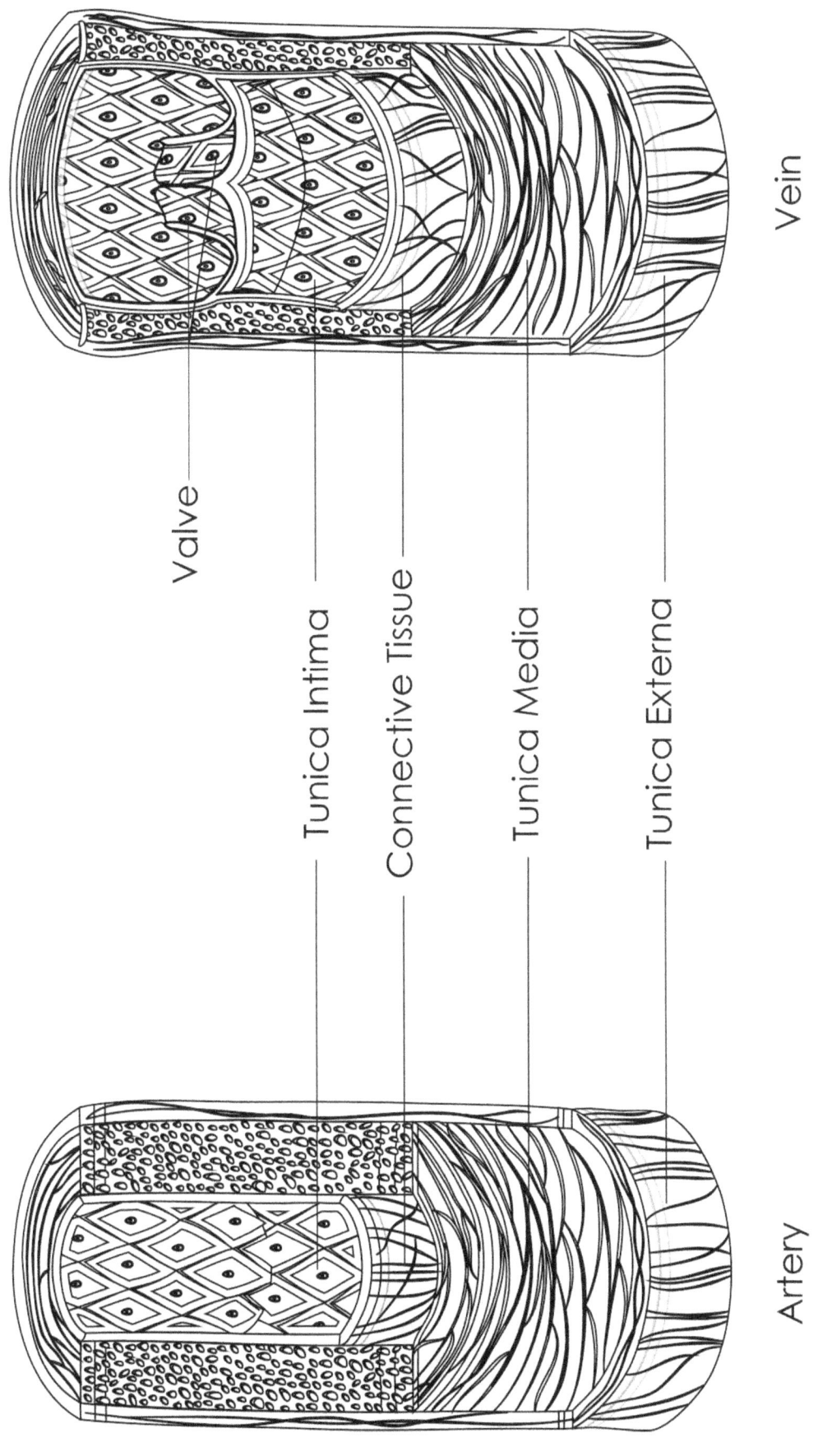

Valve

Tunica Intima

Connective Tissue

Tunica Media

Tunica Externa

Vein

Artery

ARTERY AND VEIN

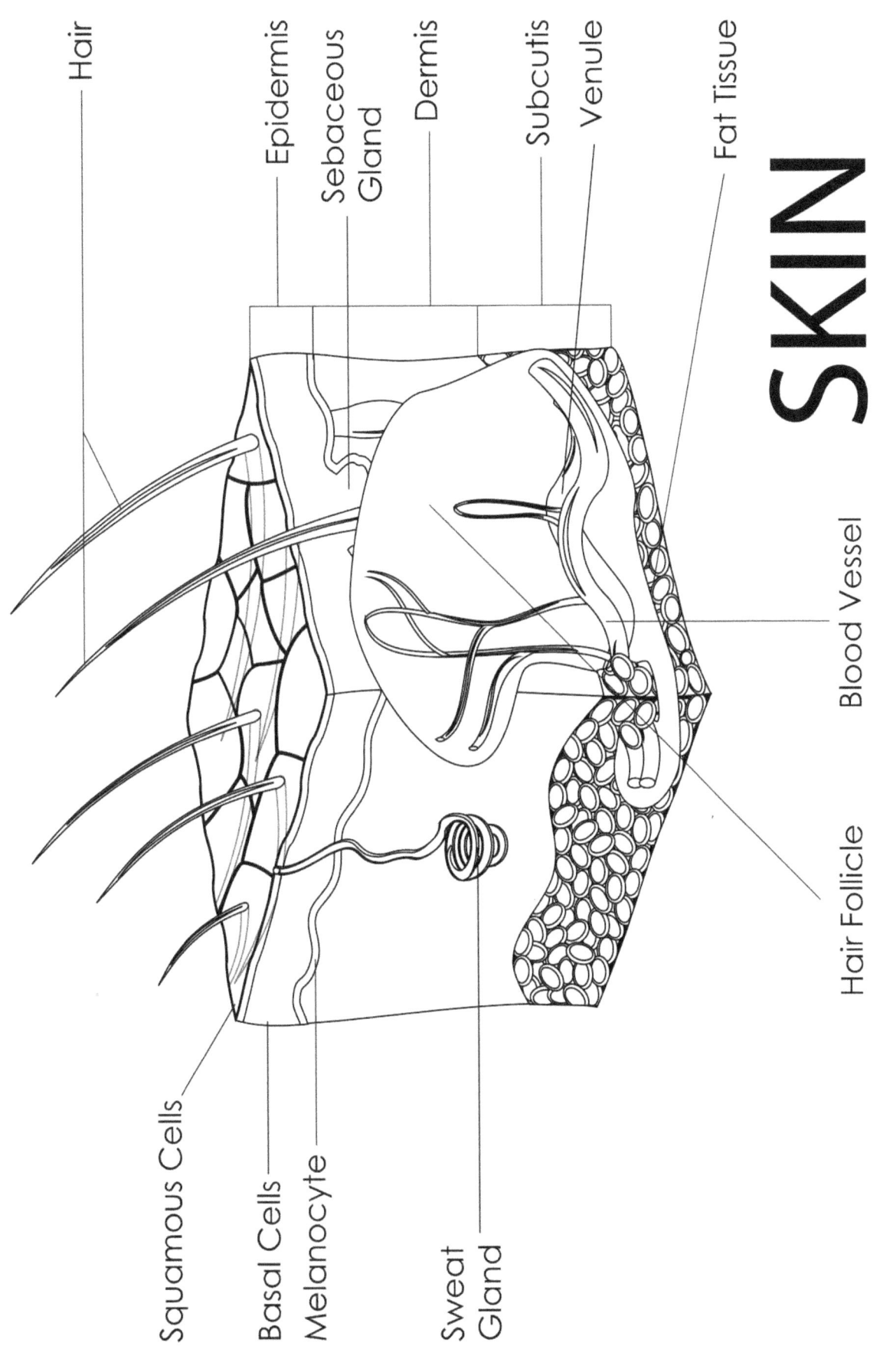

Hair

Epidermis

Sebaceous
Gland

Dermis

Subcutis

Venule

Fat Tissue

SKIN

Squamous Cells

Basal Cells

Melanocyte

Sweat
Gland

Hair Follicle

Blood Vessel

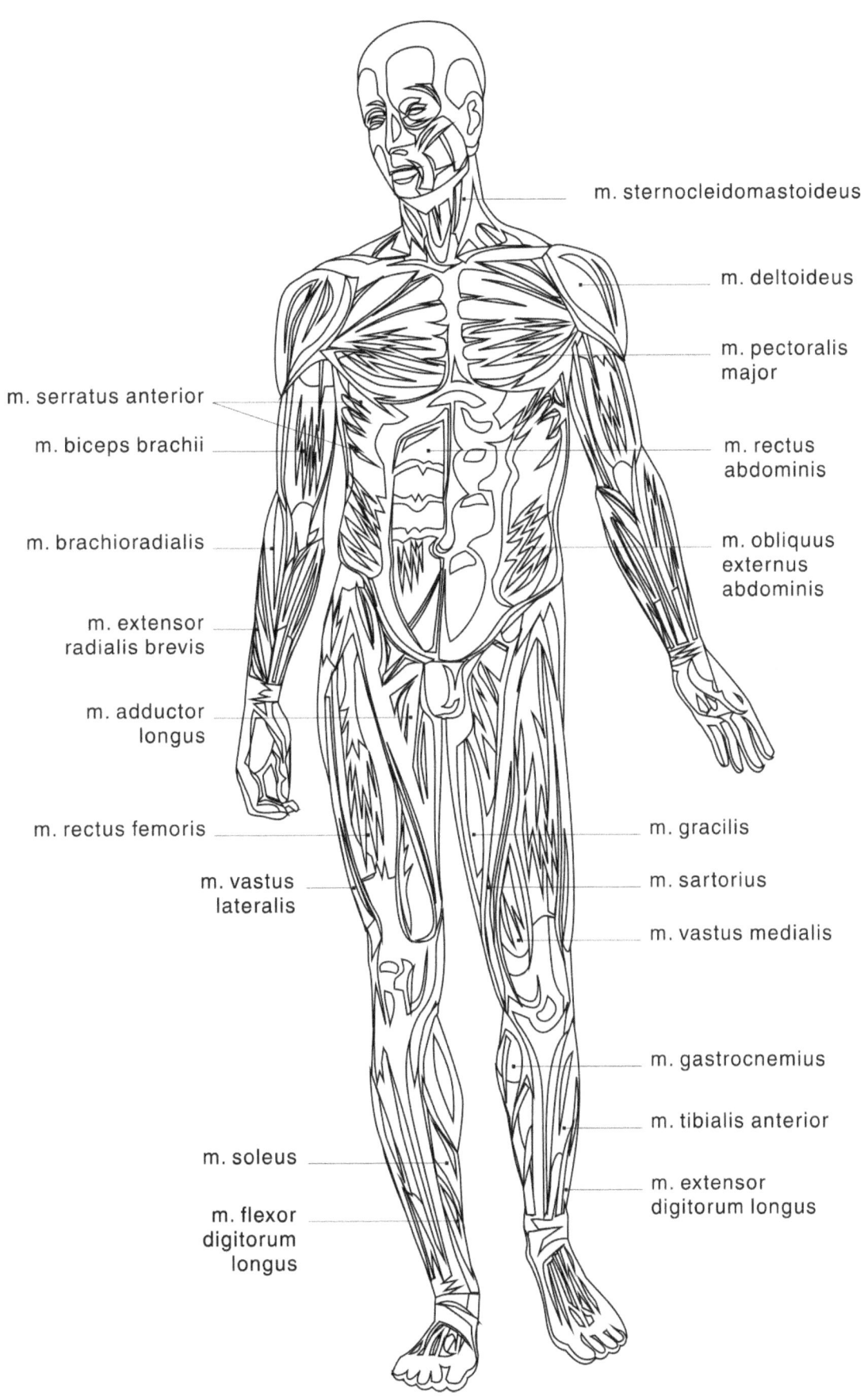

m. sternocleidomastoideus

m. deltoideus

m. pectoralis
major

m. serratus anterior

m. biceps brachii

m. rectus
abdominis

m. brachioradialis

m. obliquus
externus
abdominis

m. extensor
radialis brevis

m. adductor
longus

m. rectus femoris

m. gracilis

m. vastus
lateralis

m. sartorius

m. vastus medialis

m. gastrocnemius

m. tibialis anterior

m. soleus

m. extensor
digitorum longus

m. flexor
digitorum
longus

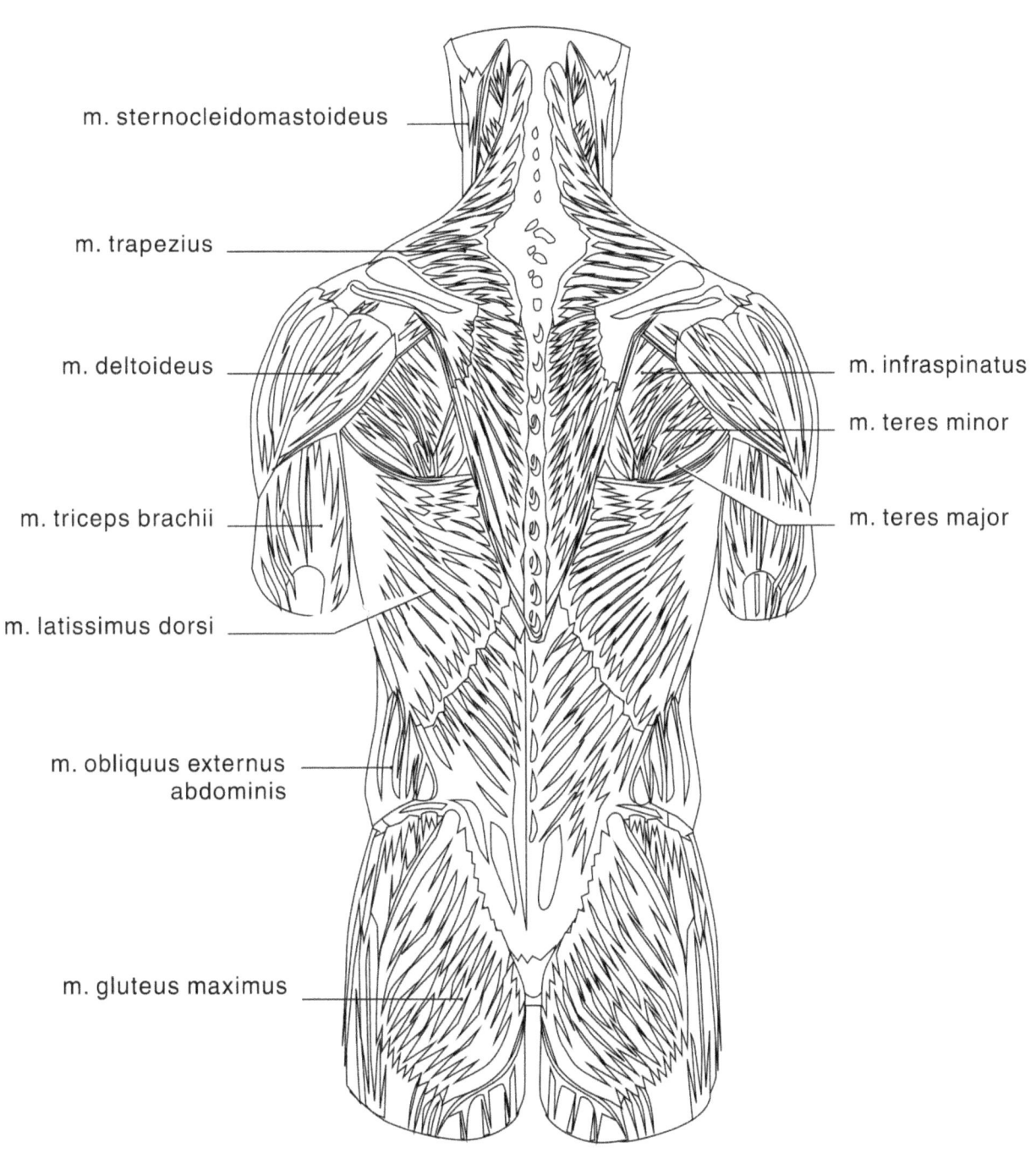

m. sternocleidomastoideus

m. trapezius

m. deltoideus

m. triceps brachii

m. latissimus dorsi

m. obliquus externus
abdominis

m. gluteus maximus

m. infraspinatus

m. teres minor

m. teres major

ORGANS

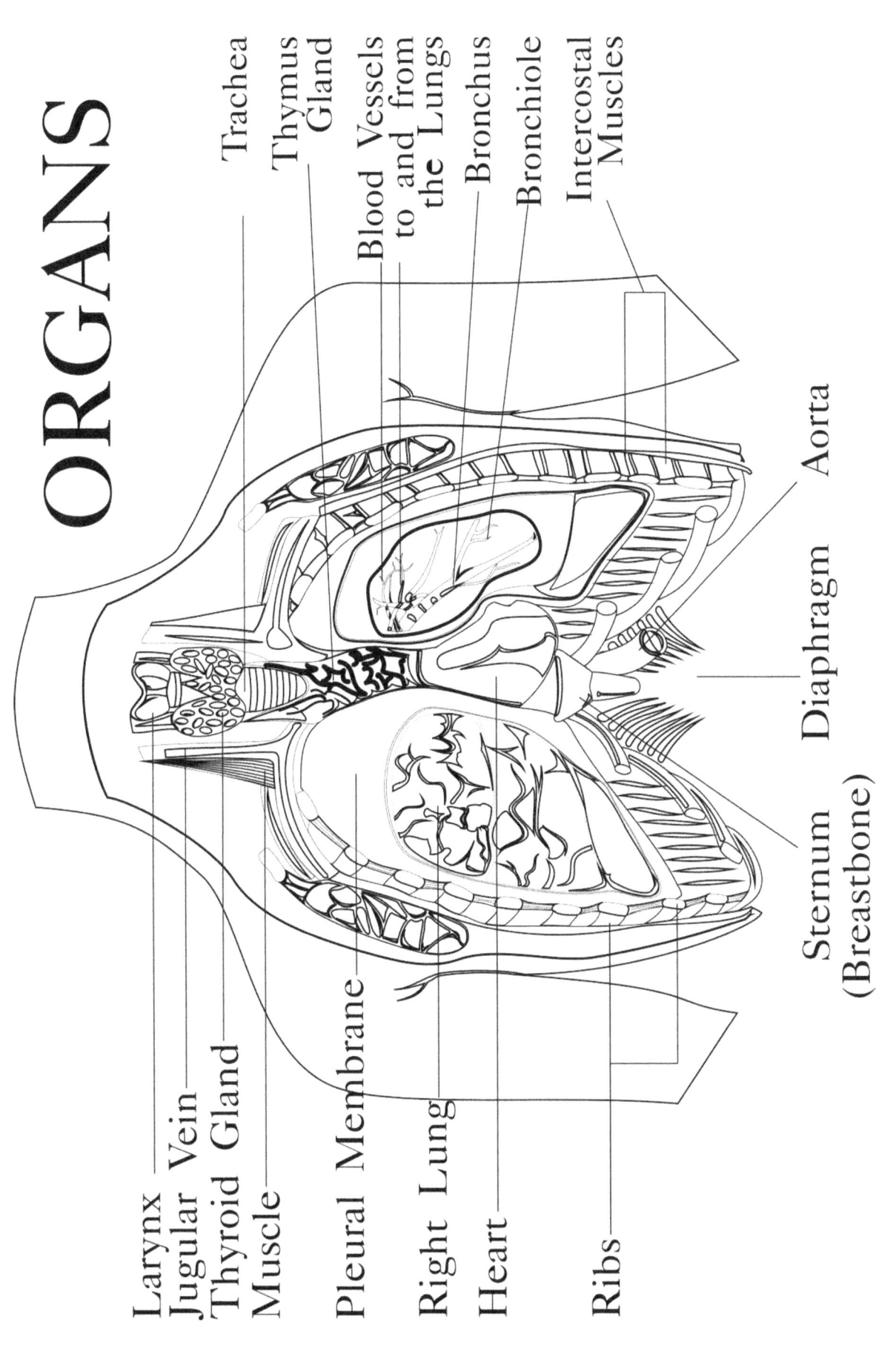

Trachea

Thymus
Gland

Blood Vessels
to and from
the Lungs

Bronchus

Bronchiole

Intercostal
Muscles

Larynx
Jugular Vein
Thyroid Gland
Muscle

Pleural Membrane

Right Lung

Heart

Ribs

Sternum
(Breastbone)

Diaphragm

Aorta

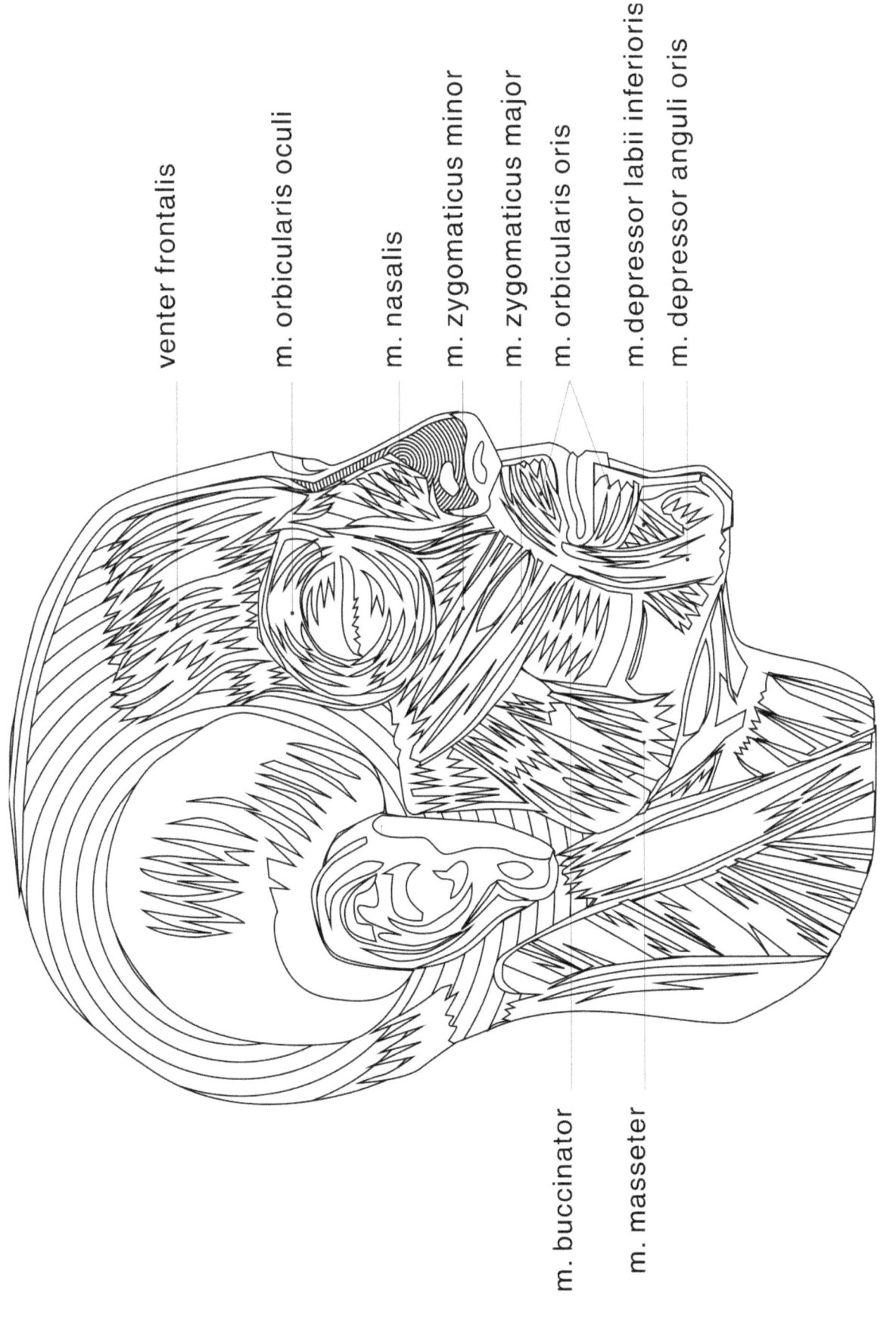

venter frontalis

m. orbicularis oculi

m. nasalis

m. zygomaticus minor

m. zygomaticus major

m. orbicularis oris

m. depressor labii inferioris

m. depressor anguli oris

m. buccinator

m. masseter